LOW FODMAP DIET COOKBOOK

From Pain to Gain - Reclaim Joy and Transform Your Gut Health with 1800 Days of Nourishing Recipes and Expert Insights into Conquering IBS and Intestinal Distress

Ella Freesia

May your health challenges be the gateways

to a deeper understanding of yourself

and the world around you.

Let your faith be bigger than your fears,

and your spirit stronger than your struggles.

This journey is part of your growth.

As the author of this book, I have dedicated immense effort and time to present you with valuable insights and knowledge. I have aimed to provide content that is both informative and inspiring, crafted with meticulous care and attention. While writing this book, I've closely adhered to the latest guidelines from experts researching the Low FODMAP diet and its effectiveness in relieving IBS symptoms, ensuring that the content and recipes are both enriching and scientifically up to date.

If you find the content of this book useful, I kindly ask you to consider leaving a review on Amazon. Your feedback not only supports my work but also assists fellow readers in discovering this book. Your thoughts and opinions are greatly appreciated and will be instrumental in shaping my future endeavors.

Thank you for your time and for choosing this book. May it serve you well.

Table of Contents

Grab your **BONUS** by scanning the **QR Code** at the end of his book

CHAPTER 1: Introduction to IBS and the Low FODMAP Diet

Imagine your stomach as a busy city, and Irritable Bowel Syndrome (IBS) is like a traffic jam causing some issues. IBS is a common tummy problem that affects the colon, which is part of your digestive system. It doesn't damage your stomach permanently, but it can make you feel uncomfortable.

Now, IBS comes with a bunch of symptoms, like tummy pain, feeling bloated (like a balloon), having gas, and dealing with either too much bathroom time (diarrhea) or not enough (constipation). It's a bit like your stomach is throwing a little party that you didn't sign up for.

Scientists aren't totally sure why IBS happens, but they think it's a mix of different things. It could be because your stomach muscles don't move things around like they should, or maybe your stomach is extra sensitive, or even because your immune system is acting a bit wonky. There's also this thing called gut microbiota, which is like the helpful bacteria in your stomach, and changes there might play a part too.

Now, here's where the Low FODMAP Diet enters the scene. FODMAPs are like special kinds of carbohydrates found in food that don't get along with some tummies. These carbs hang out in your stomach, don't get immersed properly, and end up causing a ruckus when bacteria start having a feast in your colon, making gas and other things that can make you feel not so great.

So, the Low FODMAP Diet is like a map for your meals. It helps you figure out which foods might be causing the trouble and asks you to avoid them for a little while. It's like a timeout for those pesky FODMAPs. Then, you gradually bring those foods back one by one to see which ones are causing the mischief. Once you know, you can plan your meals to keep the peace in your stomach city.

Remember, IBS might be a bit of a puzzle, but with the Low FODMAP Diet and some guidance from a healthcare friend, you can help your stomach get back to a more peaceful, easygoing state.

Overview of the Book and Digestive Health

Digestive health refers to the overall well-being and optimal functioning of the digestive system. The digestive system, also known as the gastrointestinal (GI) tract, is a complex system responsible for the breakdown of food into nutrients, absorption of these nutrients, and the elimination of waste. A healthy digestive system is essential for the proper processing of food, absorption of essential nutrients, and the elimination of waste products.

Key components of digestive health include:

1. **Efficient Digestion:** The digestive system breaks down food into smaller, absorbable components through mechanical and chemical processes. This involves the action of enzymes, stomach acid, and bile to break down proteins, carbohydrates, and fats.

2. **Nutrient Absorption:** The small intestine is primarily responsible for absorbing nutrients, such as carbohydrates, proteins, fats, vitamins, and minerals, into the bloodstream for use by the body.

3. **Gut Microbiota Balance:** The stomach and intestines are hosts to a big group of tiny living beings, commonly referred to as the gut microbiota. A balanced and diverse microbiota is essential for digestion, nutrient absorption, and immune system function.

4. **Regular Bowel Movements:** A healthy digestive system promotes regular and comfortable bowel movements. Adequate fiber intake, proper hydration, and regular physical activity contribute to regular bowel habits.

5. **Absence of Digestive Disorders:** Good digestive health involves the absence of chronic or recurring digestive disorders such as IBS, gastroesophageal reflux disease (GERD), inflammatory bowel disease (IBD), and others.

6. **Maintaining a Healthy Weight:** Digestive health is interconnected with metabolic health, and maintaining a healthy weight contributes to overall well-being.

Factors that can influence digestive health include diet, lifestyle, genetics, and environmental factors. A balanced diet rich in fiber, veggies, fruits, and whole grains, along with proper hydration, regular exercise, and stress management, can contribute to optimal digestive function.

Definition, Symptoms, and Causes of IBS, SIBO, IBD & Gluten

Irritable Bowel Syndrome (IBS)

IBS is a frequent stomach problem marked by a set of symptoms that impact the big tube in your belly called the big intestine. It is considered a functional disorder because there is no structural abnormality, but it significantly impacts the way the intestines work.

Symptoms:

• **Abdominal Pain:** IBS often causes recurrent abdominal pain or discomfort, typically relieved by bowel movements.

• **Bloating and Gas:** Excessive gas production and bloating are common symptoms.

• **Altered Bowel Habits:** IBS can lead to changes in bowel habits, including diarrhea, constipation, or a mix of both.

• **Mucus in Stool:** Some individuals with IBS may notice the presence of mucus in their stool.

Causes: The exact cause of IBS is not well understood, and it likely involves a combination of factors. Possible contributors include abnormal gastrointestinal motility, heightened visceral sensitivity, changes in gut microbiota, and alterations in the brain-gut axis. Triggers can include certain foods, stress, and hormonal changes.

Small Intestinal Bacterial Overgrowth (SIBO):

Small Intestinal Bacterial Overgrowth (SIBO) is a condition characterized by an abnormal increase in the number and/or type of bacteria in the small intestine. Normally, the small intestine has relatively fewer bacteria compared to the colon, but SIBO disrupts this balance.

Symptoms:

• **Bloating and Distension:** SIBO often leads to bloating, especially after meals.

• **Diarrhea or Constipation:** Changes in bowel habits are common.

• **Abdominal Pain:** Discomfort and pain in the abdomen are frequent symptoms.

• **Nutritional Deficiencies:** Malabsorption of nutrients can occur, leading to deficiencies.

Causes: SIBO can be caused by various factors, including impaired motility of the digestive tract, anatomical abnormalities, or conditions that affect the immune system. It can also result from previous abdominal surgeries, certain medications, or underlying conditions such as Crohn's disease.

Inflammatory Bowel Disease (IBD):

IBD refers to chronic inflammatory conditions of the digestive tract. The two main types are Crohn's disease and ulcerative colitis. Unlike IBS, IBD involves inflammation and damage to the intestinal lining.

Symptoms:

- **Abdominal Pain and Cramping:** Persistent pain and cramping are common.
- **Diarrhea with Blood:** Bloody stools and diarrhea are characteristic of IBD.
- **Weight Loss:** Loss of appetite and weight loss may occur.
- **Fatigue:** Chronic inflammation can lead to fatigue and weakness.

Causes: The precise origin of Inflammatory Bowel Disease (IBD) remains uncertain, yet it is thought to result from a complex interplay of genetic, environmental, and immune system factors. Factors such as an abnormal immune response to gut bacteria and a genetic predisposition are thought to contribute to the development of IBD.

Gluten Sensitivity and Celiac Disease:

Gluten sensitivity pertains to a state in which individuals exhibit symptoms upon consuming gluten, a protein present in wheat, barley, and rye. Celiac disease, on the other hand, is an autoimmune disorder induced by the ingestion of gluten, causing damage to the small intestine.

Symptoms:

- **Gastrointestinal Symptoms:** Both conditions can cause abdominal pain, bloating, and diarrhea.
- **Fatigue:** Chronic fatigue is a common symptom.
- **Joint Pain:** Some individuals may experience joint pain.
- **Skin Issues:** Skin rashes, such as dermatitis herpetiformis, can occur in celiac disease.

Causes: Celiac disease is an autoimmune disorder in which the immune system responds to gluten, resulting in damage to the lining of the small intestine. In contrast, gluten sensitivity, while less severe than celiac disease, is not autoimmune but can still produce comparable gastrointestinal symptoms. Genetic factors play a role in the development of both conditions.

Rome IV Diagnostic Criteria for IBS

The Rome IV criteria present as a set of diagnostic guidelines and criteria employed by healthcare professionals for the diagnosis of functional gastrointestinal disorders, such as Irritable Bowel Syndrome (IBS). These criteria were formulated by the Rome Foundation, an international organization committed to advancing the understanding and treatment of functional gastrointestinal disorders.

Diagnostic Criteria for IBS (Rome IV):

Irritable Bowel Syndrome is diagnosed based on a combination of characteristic symptoms and the absence of alarm features that may suggest a more serious underlying condition. The Rome IV criteria for IBS include the following:

1. **Recurrent Abdominal Pain:** The individual must experience abdominal pain on average almost one day per week in the last three months.

   Characteristics: The pain is associated with almost two of the following:

   - Connected to the act of defecation.
   - Linked to alterations in the frequency of bowel movements.
   - Linked to alterations in the appearance or form of stool.

2. **Onset and Duration:** The symptoms must have started almost six months prior to diagnosis.

3. **Alarm Features:**

   - Symptoms should not be explained by the presence of structural or tissue abnormalities.
   - If there are alarm features such as unexplained weight loss, blood in the stool, anemia, or a family history of certain gastrointestinal conditions, further evaluation may be necessary to rule out other disorders.

4. **Subtypes of IBS:** The Rome IV criteria further categorize IBS into subtypes based on the predominant stool pattern:

- **IBS with Diarrhea (IBS-D):** Predominant symptoms include abdominal pain and diarrhea.
- **IBS with Constipation (IBS-C):** Predominant symptoms include abdominal pain and constipation.
- **Mixed IBS (IBS-M):** Symptoms include both diarrhea and constipation.
- **Unsubtyped IBS (IBS-U):** Symptoms do not clearly fit into the above categories.

5. **Supporting Symptoms:** While not part of the primary diagnostic criteria, the Rome IV guidelines also recognize other common symptoms that may support the diagnosis of IBS. These include bloating, the sensation of incomplete evacuation, and mucus in the stool.

It's important to note that the diagnosis of IBS is primarily based on clinical evaluation and symptom patterns. The Rome IV criteria provide a standardized framework for healthcare professionals to identify and classify IBS. These criteria aim to improve consistency and accuracy in the diagnosis of functional gastrointestinal disorders, facilitating appropriate management and treatment.

Patients experiencing persistent and bothersome gastrointestinal symptoms should seek medical attention for a thorough evaluation. A healthcare professional, often a gastroenterologist, will evaluate the Rome IV criteria, gather a thorough medical history, and may conduct additional tests to exclude other conditions or confirm the diagnosis of IBS.

The Low FODMAP Diet: Origin, Research, and Benefits

The Low FODMAP Diet is a dietary approach designed to manage symptoms of irritable bowel syndrome (IBS) by reducing the intake of specific types of carbohydrates known as fermentable oligosaccharides, disaccharides, monosaccharides, and polyols (FODMAPs). Here's an overview of the diet's origin, the research supporting it, and its associated benefits.

Origin

The Low FODMAP Diet was developed by researchers at Monash University in Australia, led by Professor Peter Gibson and Dr. Susan Shepherd. The diet emerged from their research on the role of poorly immersed short-chain carbohydrates in triggering symptoms of IBS. FODMAPs, found in various foods, can ferment in the gut, leading to symptoms such as bloating, gas, abdominal pain, and altered bowel habits.

Research

The development of the Low FODMAP Diet is grounded in scientific research, particularly studies conducted by the Monash University team. The researchers conducted trials to identify high and low FODMAP foods and systematically tested their impact on individuals with IBS. The research aimed to provide evidence for the effectiveness of the diet in reducing IBS symptoms.

Benefits

• **Symptom Reduction:** The primary benefit of the Low FODMAP Diet is the reduction of IBS symptoms, including abdominal pain, bloating, gas, and irregular bowel movements. The diet is particularly helpful for individuals with IBS who have not found relief from other dietary or medical interventions.

• **Individualized Approach:** One of the strengths of the Low FODMAP Diet is its individualized nature. During the diet's implementation, individuals go through an elimination phase, followed by a reintroduction phase to identify specific FODMAPs that trigger their symptoms. This customization allows for a more targeted and sustainable approach to managing IBS.

• **Improved Quality of Life:** By effectively managing IBS symptoms, the Low FODMAP Diet has been associated with an improved quality of life for many individuals. Decreased symptoms can positively impact daily activities, social interactions, and overall well-being.

• **Supported by Dietitians:** The implementation of the Low FODMAP Diet is best done under the guidance of a registered dietitian or healthcare professional with expertise in gastrointestinal nutrition. This ensures that individuals receive proper education, support, and monitoring throughout the process.

Challenges and Considerations

• **Nutrient Adequacy:** The Low FODMAP Diet, if not followed carefully, can potentially lead to nutrient deficiencies due to restrictions on certain high-FODMAP foods that are also nutrient-dense. It is crucial for individuals to work closely with a healthcare professional to ensure nutritional adequacy.

• **Not a Long-Term Solution:** The Low FODMAP Diet is not intended as a lifelong dietary pattern. Once trigger FODMAPs are identified, individuals can reintroduce well-tolerated foods back into their diet, creating a more varied and balanced eating plan.

Lists of Foods: What to Lose and What to Choose

Foods to Avoid (High FODMAP Foods)

During the Elimination Phase of the Low FODMAP Diet, it is crucial to restrict the intake of high-FODMAP foods to alleviate symptoms associated with Irritable Bowel Syndrome (IBS). Here is a comprehensive list of high-FODMAP foods that you should avoid:

Oligosaccharides (O):

• Wheat-based products: bread, pasta, couscous, crackers, cereals

• Rye-based products: bread, crackers

• Barley-based products: bread, malt extract, some cereals

• Onions (including shallots, spring onions, and leeks)

• Garlic is one of the most concentrated sources of FODMAPs (including garlic powder and garlic-infused oils). It is added to many sauces and flavorings. In processed foods, it may be listed among the ingredients. However, garlic has many health benefits and should only be restricted in FODMAP-sensitive people.

• Legumes: lentils, chickpeas, kidney beans, black beans

Disaccharides (D):

• Lactose-containing dairy products: milk, ice cream, soft cheese, yogurt

• Some milk alternatives made from high FODMAP sources (e.g., soy milk made from whole soybeans)

Monosaccharides (M):

• High fructose fruits: apples, apricots, figs, pears, mangoes, watermelon, cherries

• Honey

• High fructose corn syrup

Polyols (P):

• Fruits: avocados, blackberries, cherries, lychees, nectarines, peaches, plums

• Artificial sweeteners: sorbitol, xylitol, mannitol, maltitol (found in sugar-free gums, mints, candies, and some processed foods)

• Some sugar alcohols used as sweeteners in certain foods and medications

Other Categories:

• Certain nuts and seeds: cashews, pistachios, chia seeds

• Certain vegetables: asparagus, Brussels sprouts, cauliflower, fennel bulbs

• Certain beverages: certain fruit juices (apple, pear), rum, certain herbal teas (chamomile)

• Processed foods: Many processed foods may contain high FODMAP components, so it's essential to check labels for additives like inulin, fructose, or high-fructose corn syrup.

A Note on High FODMAP Foods

Many foods are identified as 'High FODMAP' and often recommended to be avoided in diets for individuals with certain gastrointestinal sensitivities. However, the suitability of these foods is not always a straightforward *'black or white'* decision.

Tolerance to FODMAPs can vary greatly from person to person; some may experience discomfort from certain high FODMAP foods, while others may not. Therefore, it's beneficial to develop a personalized understanding of which specific foods trigger symptoms for you.

The Monash University FODMAP Diet App is a valuable tool in this process. It offers up-to-date information based on the latest research, helping users navigate their dietary choices more effectively. Remember, the key is to tailor your diet to your unique needs and tolerances, rather than adhering strictly to general classifications of food.

Foods to Choose (Low FODMAP Foods)

In the following tables various allowed items are listed by **category**.

If there is a specific quantity specified for a food item in the FODMAP chart, it indicates the recommended serving size that is considered low in FODMAPs. Consuming the item in that specified amount is generally understood to be safe for individuals following a low FODMAP diet, aiming to minimize the intake of fermentable oligosaccharides, disaccharides, monosaccharides, and polyols that can trigger digestive discomfort in sensitive individuals.

These quantities are determined through research and testing to establish a threshold below which most people with sensitivities do not experience symptoms. It's a guideline to help manage intake of these substances effectively.

For anyone managing a specific health condition or dietary restriction, it's always best to consult with a healthcare provider or dietitian to tailor dietary choices to individual needs.

If there is no quantity specified for certain items in the food lists, it generally means that those foods can be consumed freely without portion restrictions for maintaining a low FODMAP diet, or that the portion size does not have a significant impact on its FODMAP content within typical consumption levels. For some prepared foods, read ingredients list to verify for High FODMAP.

The list of Low FODMAP foods is updated regularly. The understanding of FODMAPs impact on conditions such as Irritable Bowel Syndrome (IBS) is continually evolving. As a result, foods are periodically reevaluated for their FODMAP content, leading to updates in the recommended lists.

Key sources for updated information on Low FODMAP foods include:

Monash University FODMAP Diet App: Monash University, a leader in FODMAP research, frequently updates its app with the latest findings. They test various foods for their FODMAP levels and update their app accordingly.

Nutritionists and Dietitians: Professionals in nutrition and dietetics keep abreast of the latest research and may update their advice to patients accordingly.

Dietary Guidelines from Health Organizations and Scientific Research and Publications.

It's important for individuals following a Low FODMAP diet to stay informed about these updates.

VEGETABLES

Item	Oz	Grams
Alfalfa		
Artichoke hearts (canned)	2.65 oz	75g
Arugula		
Banana blossom/heart		
Bamboo shoots		
Bean sprouts		
Beetroot	0.71 oz	20g
Beetroot (canned)	2.12 oz	60g
Beetroot (pickled only)		
Bell pepper (green)	2.65 oz	75g
Bell peppers (red, yellow, or orange)	1.34 oz	38g
Bok choy	2.65 oz	75g
Broccoli		
Broccolini	1.59 oz	45g
Brussel sprouts	1.34 oz	38g
Cabbage (Chinese/wombok)		
Cabbage (red or green)	2.65 oz	75g
Cabbage (red fermented)	2.47 oz	70g
Cabbage (savoy)	1.41 oz	40g
Callaloo (tinned)		
Celery	0.35 oz	10g
Chayote/Choko	2.65 oz	75g
Cho cho	2.96 oz	84g
Corn (sweet)	1.34 oz	38g
Corn (canned baby)		
Corn (canned kernels)	2.65 oz	75g
Carrot		
Eggplant	2.65 oz	75g
Endive		
Fennel bulb	1.69 oz	48g
Fennel leaves		
Gai lan		
Galangal		
Garlic shoots	1.06 oz	30g
Gourd		
Green onion/chives (green parts only)		
Jicama	4.94 oz	140g
Kale		

Item	Oz	Grams
Karela	0.53 oz	15g
Kohlrabi		
Leeks (leaves)	1.90 oz	54g
Lettuce		
Lotus root (frozen)	2.65 oz	75g
Mushrooms (champignons canned)	2.65 oz	75g
Mushrooms (oyster type)		
Okra	2.65 oz	75g
Olives (black and green)		
Onions (large pickled only)	1.59 oz	45g
Peas (canned)	1.59 oz	45g
Peas (snap)	0.49 oz	14g
Peas (snow)	0.56 oz	16g
Parsnip		
Potatoes		
Sweet potato	2.65 oz	75g
Pumpkin (canned)	2.65 oz	75g
Radish		
Rutabega/Swede	2.65 oz	75g
Seaweed/nori		
Silverbeet		
Snakebean/yardlong	2.65 oz	75g
Spinach		
Squash (butternut)	1.59 oz	45g
Squash (kabocha, pattypan, & spaghetti)		
Swiss chard		
Taro	2.65 oz	75g
Tomatillo	2.65 oz	75g
Tomatoes (cherry)	1.59 oz	45g
Tomatoes (common)	2.29 oz	65g
Tomatoes (roma)	1.69 oz	48g
Tomatoes (canned)	3.24 oz	92g
Tomatoes (sun-dried)	0.28 oz	8g
Turnip/Rutabega	2.65 oz	75g
Water chestnuts		
Witlof		
Yam	2.65 oz	75g
Zucchini	2.29 oz	65g

FRUITS

Item	Oz	Grams
Avocado (1/8 whole)	1.06 oz	30g
Banana unripe		
Banana ripe with brown spots (1/3 medium fruit)	1.23 oz	35g
Banana dried (15 chips)	1.06 oz	30g
Blueberries		
Boysenberry (5 berries)	0.42 oz	12g
Breadfruit		
Cantaloupe melon (3/4 C)	4.23 oz	120g
Clementine		
Coconut dried shredded (1/2 C)	1.06 oz	30g
Coconut fresh (2/3 C)	2.26 oz	64g
Cranberries dried (1 Tbsp)	0.53 oz	15g
Cranberries raw (1/2 C)	1.76 oz	50g
Cumquats		
Currants (1 Tbsp)	0.46 oz	13g
Dates dried (5 dates)	1.06 oz	30g
Dates medjool (1 date)	0.71 oz	20g
Dragon fruit		
Durian		
Goji berries (3 tsp)	0.35 oz	10g
Grapes (6)	0.99 oz	28g
Grapefruit (1/3 C)	2.82 oz	80g
Honeydew melon (1/2 C)	3.17 oz	90g
Jackfruit canned (1/3C)	1.59 oz	45g

Item	Oz	Grams
Kiwi (2 small)	5.29 oz	150g
Lemon juice		
Lime juice		
Longan (2.5 longans)	0.88 oz	25g
Lychee (3 lychees)	1.06 oz	30g
Mandarins		
Mango (1/5 C)	1.41 oz	40g
Mangosteen (2)	1.76 oz	50g
Nectarine white (1/2 fruit)	2.12 oz	60g
Orange navel		
Papaya yellow or green		
Passionfruit (2 fruits)	1.62 oz	46g
Paw paw (1 C)	4.94 oz	140g
Peach yellow (1/4 C)	1.06 oz	30g
Pear only prickly type		
Persimmon (3/4 C)		67g
Pineapple (1 C)	4.94 oz	140g
Pomegranate seeds (1/4 C)	1.59 oz	45g
Raisins regular (1 Tbsp)	0.46 oz	13g
Raspberry (1/3 C)	2.05 oz	58g
Rhubarb		
Rambutan (3)	1.69 oz	48g
Star fruit/Carambola		
Strawberries (5)	2.29 oz	65g
Tamarind (4)	0.28 oz	8g

PROTEINS

Item	Oz	Grams
All Meat/Poultry/Fish/Eggs		
Egg replacer	N/A	1 tsp
Nuts tigernuts	0.71 oz	20g
Beans canned adzuki / black / butter / chickpeas / kidney	1.41 oz	40g
Beans cannellini canned	2.68 oz	76g
Beans chana dahl & urid dahl	1.62 oz	46g
Lentils red/green boiled	0.81 oz	23g
Nuts almonds	0.42 oz	12g
Nuts peanut butter	1.76 oz	50g
Nuts pecan	0.71 oz	20g
Beans edamame	3.17 oz	90g
Nuts almond butter	0.71 oz	20g
Nuts pine	0.49 oz	14g
Nuts walnuts	1.06 oz	30g
Beans lima boiled	1.38 oz	39g

Item	Oz	Grams
Nuts brazil	1.41 oz	40g
Seeds chia	0.85 oz	24g
Beans mung boiled	1.87 oz	53g
Nuts chestnuts	2.96 oz	84g
Seeds flax	0.53 oz	15g
Beans mung sprouted	3.35 oz	95g
Nuts hazelnuts	0.53 oz	15g
Seeds hemp	0.71 oz	20g
Beans pinto canned/refried	1.59 oz	45g
Nuts macadamia	1.41 oz	40g
Seeds poppy	0.85 oz	24g
Seeds pumpkin	0.81 oz	23g
Seeds sesame	0.39 oz	11g
Seeds sunflower	0.21 oz	6g
Soy mince	1.45 oz	41g
Tofu firm	5.64 oz	160g
Tempeh	3.53 oz	100g

GRAINS

Item	Oz	Grams
Amaranth puffed	0.35 oz	10g
Almond meal	0.85 oz	24g
Arrowroot		
Bran oat	0.78 oz	22g
Bran rice	0.56 oz	16g
Breadcrumbs panko	2.65 oz	75g
Buckwheat grouts cooked	4.76 oz	135g
Corn meal/maize & polenta		
Corn tortillas	2.47 oz	70g
Gluten-free breads cookies crackers pasta noodles etc. (without added FODMAPs)		
Some gluten-free flours (arrowroot buckwheat cassava corn green banana millet quinoa rice sieved spelt sorghum teff yam)		
Kelp noodles	3.99 oz	113g

Item	Oz	Grams
Millet kernels cooked	4.41 oz	125g
Millet bread	1.98 oz	56g
Oats rolled & flakes	1.76 oz	50g
Oat groats	2.12 oz	60g
Pretzels	0.85 oz	24g
Popcorn		
Quinoa red/ white/ black/ flakes/ pasta		
Pearl barley sprouted	3.53 oz	100g
Rice white/ brown/ red/ crackers/ flakes /noodles		
Rice wild	4.94 oz	140g
Rice cakes	0.99 oz	28g
Sago	5.64 oz	160g
Samp cooked	5.22 oz	148g
Sorghum		
Sourdough traditional long ferment no yeast wheat or spelt flour (2 slices)		
Starches corn/ potato/ tapioca		

DAIRY AND ALTERNATIVES

Item	Oz	Grams
Butter		
Hard cheeses (brie, camembert, cheddar, Colby, feta, goat, Havarti, mozzarella, pecorino, Swiss)		
Soft cheeses (cottage, cream, haloumi, paneer, quark, ricotta)	1.41 oz	40g
Soy cheese	1.41 oz	40g
Cream	1.41 oz	40g
Cream whipped	2.12 oz	60g
Cream sour	1.41 oz	40g

Item	Oz	Grams
Coconut cream	2.12 oz	60g
Milk hemp		1/2 C
Milk macadamia		1 C
Coconut yogurt	4.41 oz	125g
Milk oat		1/2 C
Lactose-free milk and products		
Milk almond		1 C
Milk coconut		1/2 C
Milk canned coconut	2.12 oz	60g
Milk quinoa		1 C
Milk rice		3/4 C
Milk soy protein		1 C

SWEETENERS

Item	Oz	Grams
Agave syrup	0.18 oz	5g
Artificial sweeteners (aspartame, saccharin, sucralose, stevia)		
Coconut sugar	0.14 oz	4g
Glucose		
Golden syrup	0.25 oz	7g
Honey	0.25 oz	7g
Honey clover	0.11 oz	3g

Item	Oz	Grams
Malt extract	0.46 oz	13g
Maple syrup		
Molasses	0.18 oz	5g
Rice malt syrup		
Regular corn syrup		
Sorghum syrup	0.71 oz	20g
Sugar / sucrose (brown, cane, palm, raw, white)		
Treacle coconut syrup	0.49 oz	14g

BEVERAGES

Item	Oz	Grams
Aloe drink	2.26 oz	64g
Beer	12.68 oz	375 mL
Coconut water	3.38 oz	100 mL
Coffee		
Cranberry juice	5.41 oz	160 mL
Espresso		
Pops/soda		
Kombucha	6.09 oz	180 mL
Kvass		1 C
Some spirits (gin, tequila, vodka, whisky)		
Teas strongly infused (buchu, epazote, green,		

Item	Oz	Grams
honeybush, licorice, peppermint, rooibos / red, white)		
Teas weakly infused (black, chai, chrysanthemum, dandelion)		
Tomato juice	3.04 oz	90g
Water regular/sparkling		
Wheatgrass powder		1 tsp
Wine red / sparkling / sweet / white	5.07 oz	150 mL

OTHER FOOD

Items	Oz	Grams
Achiote / Annatti paste	1 Tbsp	20g
Agar		7g
Asafetida powder		
Bay Leaves	1 leaf	
Barbeque sauce	2 Tbsp	
Black pepper sauce	1 Tbsp	15g
Broth/stock		
Cacao & cocoa powder	2 heaped tsp	8g
Carob powder	1 heaped tsp	6g
Capers	1 tbsp	8g
Caviar dip	1/2 Tbsp	10g
Chestnut cream	1 Tbsp	19g
Chimichurri sauce	2 Tbsp	40g
Chives		
Chocolate (dark <30g; white <25g; milk <20g)		
Chutney	1 Tbsp	25g
Coconut aminos	1 tsp	5g
Coconut cream	1/4 C	60g
Coconut jam	1/2 Tbsp	11g
Corn relish	1 Tbsp	20g
Creamer powder	2 tsp	3g
Eggplant dip	2 Tbsp	40g
Egg replacer	1 tbsp	6g
Fish sauce	1 Tbsp	44g
Ginger root		
Gherkins in vinegar		
Habanero sauce	1 tsp	10g
Herbs		
Horseradish	2 Tbsp	42g
Jam strawberry/raspberry	2 Tbsp	40g
Jello/instant jelly		
Kelp noodles	1 C	113g
Ketchup	1 Tbsp	15g
Licorice black		45g
Maca powder	1 tsp	
Marmalade	2 Tbsp	40g
Matcha	1 tsp	
Mayonnaise		

Items	Oz	Grams
Mint jelly & sauce	1 Tbsp	20g
Miso paste*	1 Tbsp	12g
Mustard	1 Tbsp	
Nutritional yeast flakes	1 Tbsp	16g
Oils (avocado, coconut, olive, sunflower, etc.)		
Oils infused		
Oyster sauce	1 Tbsp	20g
Pea protein powder	2 Tbsp	40g
Peanut butter	2 Tbsp	
Pickles		
Potato chips		
Quince paste	1/2 Tbsp	13g
Relish	1 Tbsp	20g
Remoulade sauce	2 Tbsp	
Salsa	2 Tbsp	30g
Shrimp paste	2 tsp	10g
Soy sauce	2 Tbsp	42g
Spirulina		
Spices		
Sriracha	1 tsp	5g
Sweet and sour sauce	2 Tbsp	44g
Tahini	2 Tbsp	30g
Tamarind paste	1/2 Tbsp	11g
Tomato juice	1/3 C	90g
Tomato paste	2 Tbsp	28g
Tomato sauce	1/2 C	
Vanilla bean pods & extract/essence		
Vegemite	1 tsp	5g
Verjuice		
Vinegars apple cider / malt / red wine / rice wine	2 tbsp	42g
Vinegar balsamic	1 Tbsp	21g
Vinegar white		
Worcestershire sauce	2 Tbsp	42g
Wheatgrass powder	1 tsp	3g
Xantham gum		

CHAPTER 2: Mastering Your Low FODMAP Journey

Embarking on the Low FODMAP journey is a transformative process, and understanding its three crucial phases—Elimination, Reintroduction, and Personalization—is key to managing Irritable Bowel Syndrome (IBS) effectively.

3-Phase Journey: Elimination, Reintroduction and Personalization Phases

The Low FODMAP Diet stands as a testament to the evolving field of nutritional science, providing a targeted and evidence-based approach to managing Irritable Bowel Syndrome (IBS). At its core, the diet recognizes the impact of fermentable carbohydrates—FODMAPs—on digestive health and aims to empower individuals to navigate their dietary choices with precision. The diet involves three main phases:

1. **Elimination Phase:** During this phase, high-FODMAP foods are restricted from the diet for a specific period, usually 2 to 6 weeks. This helps identify which FODMAPs trigger symptoms for an individual.

2. **Reintroduction Phase:** In this phase, high-FODMAP foods are systematically reintroduced one at a time to identify which specific carbohydrates are causing symptoms. This helps customize the diet based on individual tolerance.

3. **Maintenance Phase:** Once trigger FODMAPs are identified, the individual follows a modified diet that limits only the specific carbohydrates that trigger symptoms, allowing for a more varied and personalized diet.

It's essential to emphasize that the Low FODMAP Diet is not intended as a long-term solution. Instead, it serves as a valuable tool for uncovering and managing specific triggers for IBS symptoms. In tandem with the dietary modifications, maintaining a balanced and nutritionally adequate diet remains paramount, safeguarding overall health and nutritional well-being.

The Low FODMAP Diet transcends a generic approach to dietary management, ushering in a new era where individuals actively participate in understanding and navigating the intricate relationship between their food choices and digestive health.

The Importance of Guidance by a Dietitian

Embarking on the Low FODMAP journey to manage Irritable Bowel Syndrome (IBS) is a transformative process, and the guidance of a registered dietitian specializing in gastrointestinal health is paramount for several compelling reasons.

4. **Expertise in Nutritional Science:** Dietitians possess extensive education and training in nutritional science. Their understanding of the intricacies of the Low FODMAP Diet, including the specific types of carbohydrates to be restricted during the elimination phase and the systematic reintroduction of FODMAPs, is crucial. Their expertise ensures that individuals receive accurate and up-to-date information, promoting effective symptom management and nutritional well-being.

5. **Personalized Approach:** Every individual's response to FODMAPs is unique. A dietitian plays a pivotal role in tailoring the Low FODMAP journey to the specific needs and sensitivities of each person. Through careful assessment, the dietitian helps create a personalized plan that addresses individual triggers, nutritional requirements, and lifestyle considerations. This personalized approach maximizes the effectiveness of the diet while minimizing potential nutritional deficiencies.

6. **Interpretation of Symptoms:** The reintroduction phase, where FODMAPs are systematically reintroduced to identify triggers, requires careful observation and interpretation of symptoms. A dietitian guides individuals through this process, helping them understand the subtle nuances of their body's responses. This professional insight is invaluable in distinguishing between various symptoms and accurately identifying specific FODMAP triggers, facilitating a more precise and individualized dietary plan.

7. **Nutritional Adequacy:** Balancing the restriction of high FODMAP foods with nutritional adequacy is a delicate task. Dietitians are equipped to ensure that individuals following the Low FODMAP Diet receive the essential nutrients needed for overall health. They provide guidance on suitable alternatives, supplementation if necessary, and strategies to maintain a well-rounded and nourishing diet despite the limitations imposed by the FODMAP restrictions.

8. **Emotional Support and Education:** The Low FODMAP journey can be emotionally challenging, impacting one's relationship with food and overall well-being. Dietitians offer not only nutritional guidance but also emotional support. They educate individuals about the principles of the diet, help manage expectations, and empower them with the knowledge and skills needed to navigate social situations, dining out, and unexpected challenges.

When to Seek Help and How to build a Support System

Navigating the Low FODMAP journey for managing Irritable Bowel Syndrome (IBS) can be both empowering and challenging. Knowing when to seek help and establishing a robust support system are essential elements for a successful and sustainable journey.

When to Seek Help

• **Persistent or Worsening Symptoms:** If IBS symptoms persist or worsen despite following the Low FODMAP Diet, seeking professional guidance is crucial. A healthcare professional, particularly a registered dietitian with expertise in gastrointestinal health, can assess the situation and make necessary adjustments.

• **Difficulty Interpreting Responses:** The reintroduction phase, where specific FODMAP groups are systematically reintroduced, can be complex. If individuals find it challenging to interpret their body's responses accurately, a dietitian can provide insights, helping distinguish between various symptoms and identify specific triggers.

• **Nutritional Concerns:** Individuals may face nutritional concerns due to the restrictions imposed by the Low FODMAP Diet. A dietitian can address these concerns, ensuring nutritional adequacy, and may recommend appropriate supplements if needed.

• **Impact on Mental Health:** The emotional toll of managing dietary restrictions and symptoms can be significant. If the Low FODMAP journey impacts mental health or leads to anxiety around food, seeking help from a mental health professional or counselor is essential.

Building a Support System

• **Share Your Journey:** Communicate openly with friends and family about your Low FODMAP journey. Sharing your experiences fosters understanding and encourages a supportive environment.

• **Online Communities and Support Groups:** Joining online communities and support groups dedicated to IBS and the Low FODMAP Diet provides a platform to connect with others facing similar challenges. Sharing insights, tips, and encouragement can be invaluable.

• **Local Support Groups:** Explore local IBS support groups where you can connect with individuals in your community facing similar experiences. These groups often organize meetings, events, or even cooking sessions, providing a sense of community.

• **Communication with Healthcare Providers:** Regular check-ins with healthcare professionals, including dietitians, gastroenterologists, and primary care providers, ensure ongoing support, guidance, and adjustments to the dietary plan based on your evolving needs.

3 Keys Pillars: Kitchen Prep, Meal Planning, and Dining Out

Successfully navigating the Low FODMAP journey involves incorporating three foundational pillars—Kitchen Prep, Meal Planning, and Dining Out. These pillars present as essential elements in maintaining a well-balanced and sustainable approach to managing Irritable Bowel Syndrome (IBS) symptoms.

Kitchen Prep

A well-prepared kitchen is the cornerstone of the Low FODMAP journey. Key aspects of Kitchen Prep include:

• **Stocking Low FODMAP Staples:** Maintain a supply of Low FODMAP pantry staples and components. This ensures you have a foundation for creating flavorful and compliant meals.

• **Labeling High and Low FODMAP Items:** Clearly label foods in your kitchen as high or low FODMAP to streamline decision-making and avoid unintentional consumption of trigger foods.

• **Reading Food Labels:** Develop the habit of reading food labels meticulously. Look out for hidden FODMAPs in packaged products, such as onion or garlic powder.

Meal Planning

Thoughtful Meal Planning is essential for creating a varied and nutritionally balanced diet while adhering to the Low FODMAP principles:

• **Weekly Meal Plans:** Plan your meals for the week, incorporating a diverse range of low FODMAP foods. This helps avoid monotony and ensures a mix of nutrients.

• **Preparing Snacks and Meals in Advance:** Proactively prepare Low FODMAP snacks and meals in advance, especially during busy periods. This reduces the likelihood of resorting to less suitable food options.

• **Rotating Recipes:** Keep your meal plans dynamic by rotating recipes. This maintains interest, prevents culinary fatigue, and allows you to explore the vast array of Low FODMAP-friendly dishes.

Dining Out

Successfully navigating dining out experiences involves strategic decision-making and effective communication:

• **Communication with Restaurants:** Communicate your dietary needs with restaurant staff. Many establishments are willing to accommodate specific requests or modify dishes to meet Low FODMAP criteria.

• **Opting for Simple Dishes:** Choose simple, whole food-based dishes when dining out. These are more likely to be Low FODMAP and reduce the risk of hidden triggers.

• **Being Proactive:** Take a proactive approach to dining out. Research restaurant menus in advance, inquire about preparation methods, and plan your choices ahead of time.

How to Integrate Recipes into a Meal Plan

Creating a well-rounded Low FODMAP meal plan involves thoughtful integration of recipes to ensure variety, nutritional balance, and adherence to dietary restrictions:

Recipe Selection

• Choose recipes that feature Low FODMAP components, emphasizing a mix of protein sources, low FODMAP vegetables, and suitable grains or carbohydrates.

• Experiment with different cuisines to maintain diversity in flavors and textures.

• Adapt favorite recipes to be Low FODMAP by substituting high FODMAP components with suitable alternatives.

Balanced Meals

• Ensure each meal includes a combination of essential components, such as protein, low FODMAP vegetables, and appropriate carbohydrates.

• Consider portion sizes to avoid overconsumption of FODMAPs while meeting nutritional needs.

• Aim for a balance of macronutrients and micronutrients in each meal to support overall well-being.

Planning for Success

• Create a weekly meal plan that incorporates a range of Low FODMAP recipes. This helps avoid monotony and ensures a diverse nutrient intake.

• Prepare a shopping list based on the planned recipes to streamline grocery shopping.

• Monitor symptoms and adjust the meal plan as needed, allowing for flexibility and adaptation based on individual responses.

Ready to start preparing you recipes? A last word..

We're all set to begin exploring and enjoying the flavors of Low FODMAP recipes, featuring delicious natural ingredients. Before we dive in, please take a moment to thoroughly read the following recommendations to fully comprehend and embrace them.

The following recipes have been meticulously analyzed for their content of Low FODMAP ingredients, while striving to maintain their deliciousness and ease of preparation. However, it's important to recognize that no single recipe is ideal for everyone. Individual sensitivities to certain ingredients vary widely. Therefore, it is highly recommended to always review the ingredients and replace those that may not be well-tolerated. The 180 recipes provided here are intended as suggestions, offering readers the freedom to experiment with alternative ingredients that may be more beneficial and cause no discomfort. Remember, no recipe is more important than a person's awareness of their own symptoms. Listening to your body is crucial to understanding what makes you feel good and what doesn't.

NOTE to Recipes quantities:

A Global Kitchen Measurement TABLE is reported at the end of Chapter 4

CHAPTER 3: Low FODMAP Living: 180 Recipes and Meal Plans

NOTE: For any recipe, an asterisk (*) beside an ingredient indicates it should be eaten moderately. Confirm permissible quantities via the Monash University FODMAP Diet app or similar resources as reported in Chapter 4.

Breakfast Recipes

1 - Scrambled Eggs with Spinach and Tomatoes

Preparation time: 5 min.

Cooking time: 10 min.

Servings: 2

Ingredients:

- 4 eggs
- 1 cup fresh spinach, hand-torn
- 1 cup cherry tomatoes, divided*
- Salt and pepper as required

Directions:

1. In your container, whisk the eggs then season with salt and pepper.

2. Heat a non-stick griddle over medium heat.

3. Put the hand-torn spinach and cherry tomatoes to the griddle then cook until spinach wilts and tomatoes soften.

4. Pour the whisked eggs over the vegetables and carefully scramble until eggs are fully cooked.

5. Present instantly.

Per serving: Calories: 180 kcal; Fat: 12g; Carbs: 5g; Protein: 14g; Fiber: 2g; Sodium: 320mg

2 - Quinoa Breakfast Bowl with Berries

Preparation time: 10 min.

Cooking time: 15 min.

Servings: 2

Ingredients:

- 1 cup quinoa, washed
- 2 cups lactose-free almond milk
- 1 cup Low FODMAP mixed berries (e.g., blueberries)
- 2 tbsps maple syrup
- Chopped nuts (elective, for topping)

Directions:

1. In a saucepot, blend quinoa and almond milk. Bring to a boil, then reduce the heat. then simmer until quinoa is cooked and liquid is immersed.

2. Split the cooked quinoa into two containers.

3. Top with mixed berries and drizzle with maple syrup.

4. Optional: Garnish with chopped nuts for added texture.

Per serving: Calories: 320 kcal; Fat: 6g; Carbs: 60g; Protein: 8g; Fiber: 6g; Sodium: 120mg

3 - Smoked Salmon and Avocado Wrap

Preparation time: 10 min.

Cooking time: 0 min.

Servings: 2

Ingredients:

- 4 gluten-free wraps
- 6 oz smoked salmon
- 1 ripe avocado, carved
- Fresh dill (elective, for garnish)

Directions:

1. Lay out the wraps and divide the smoked salmon and avocado slices among them.

2. Optional: Garnish with fresh dill.

3. Roll up the wraps and slice in half.

Per serving: Calories: 400 kcal; Fat: 20g; Carbs: 30g; Protein: 25g; Fiber: 8g; Sodium: 900mg

4 - Blueberry Oat Pancakes

Preparation time: 15 min.

Cooking time: 10 min.

Servings: 2

Ingredients:

- 1 cup gluten-free oats
- 1 ripe banana, mashed
- 2 eggs
- 1/2 cup lactose-free almond milk
- 1/2 cup blueberries
- Maple syrup for drizzling

Directions:

1. In a blender, blend oats, banana, eggs, and almond milk. Blend until smooth.

2. Gently wrap in the blueberries.

3. Heat a non-stick griddle over medium heat. and ladle the batter to form pancakes.

4. Cook the food until bubbles appear on the surface, then turn it over and continue cooking the other side.

5. Present with a drizzle of maple syrup.

Per serving: Calories: 350 kcal; Fat: 12g; Carbs: 50g; Protein: 12g; Fiber: 7g; Sodium: 180mg

5 - Chia Seed Pudding with Kiwi

Preparation time: 5 min. (plus overnight chilling)

Cooking time: 0 min.

Servings: 2

Ingredients:

- 1/4 cup chia seeds
- 1 cup lactose-free almond milk
- 1 tbsp maple syrup
- 2 kiwis, skinned and carved

Directions:

1. In your container, mix chia seeds, almond milk, and maple syrup.

2. Stir well and put in the fridge overnight or almost 4 hrs until the solution thickens.

3. Split the pudding into two containers and top with carved kiwi.

Per serving: Calories: 220 kcal; Fat: 10g; Carbs: 28g; Protein: 6g; Fiber: 12g; Sodium: 80mg

6 - Banana Almond Butter Smoothie

Preparation time: 5 min.

Cooking time: 0 min.

Servings: 2

Ingredients:

- 2 ripe bananas*
- 2 tbsps almond butter
- 1 cup lactose-free yogurt
- 1 cup ice cubes
- 1 tbsp chia seeds (elective)

Directions:

1. In a blender, blend ripe bananas, almond butter, lactose-free yogurt, and ice cubes.

2. Blend until smooth.

3. Optional: Stir in chia seeds for added texture.

Per serving: Calories: 280 kcal; Fat: 12g; Carbs: 35g; Protein: 8g; Fiber: 6g; Sodium: 60mg

7 - Zucchini and Feta Omelet

Preparation time: 10 min.

Cooking time: 10 min.

Servings: 2

Ingredients:

- 4 eggs
- 1 zucchini, grated*
- 1/2 cup crumbled lactose-free feta cheese
- Salt and pepper as required
- Fresh parsley for garnish

Directions:

1. In your container, whisk the eggs then season with salt and pepper.

2. Heat a non-stick griddle over medium heat.

3. Include grated zucchini to the griddle then cook until softened.

4. Pour the whisked eggs over the zucchini then crumble feta cheese on top.

5. Cook until the eggs are set, then wrap the omelet in half.

6. Garnish with fresh parsley and present.

Per serving: Calories: 280 kcal; Fat: 20g; Carbs: 6g; Protein: 18g; Fiber: 2g; Sodium: 480mg

8 - Cinnamon Raisin Overnight Oats

Preparation time: 10 min. (plus overnight chilling)

Cooking time: 0 min.

Servings: 2

Ingredients:

- 1 cup gluten-free oats
- 1 cup lactose-free almond milk
- 1 tbsp maple syrup
- 1/4 cup raisins*
- 1/2 tsp ground cinnamon

Directions:

1. In your container, blend oats, almond milk, maple syrup, raisins, and cinnamon.

2. Stir well and put in the fridge overnight.

3. Split the overnight oats into two containers and present.

Per serving: Calories: 250 kcal; Fat: 6g; Carbs: 44g; Protein: 6g; Fiber: 5g; Sodium: 80mg

9 - Greek Yogurt Parfait with Strawberries

Preparation time: 5 min.

Cooking time: 0 min.

Servings: 2

Ingredients:

- 2 cups lactose-free Greek yogurt
- 1 cup strawberries, carved*
- 2 tbsps sunflower seeds (elective)
- 1 tbsp maple syrup (elective)

Directions:

1. In two glasses or containers, layer Greek yogurt and carved strawberries.

2. Optional: Drizzle each layer with a bit of maple syrup for sweetness.

3. Top with sunflower seeds for added crunch.

4. Repeat the layers and finish with a strawberry on top.

Per serving: Calories: 250 kcal; Fat: 10g; Carbs: 25g; Protein: 15g; Fiber: 4g; Sodium: 80mg

10 - Polenta and Vegetable Breakfast Skillet

Preparation time: 10 min.

Cooking time: 15 min.

Servings: 2

Ingredients:

- 1 cup cooked polenta, carved
- 1 zucchini, cubed*
- 1 red bell pepper, cubed**
- 2 tbsps olive oil
- Salt and pepper as required
- Fresh parsley for garnish

Directions:

1. Heat olive oil on your griddle over medium heat.

2. Include cubed zucchini and bell pepper, sauté until softened.

3. Include carved polenta to the griddle then cook until fully heated.

4. Season with salt and pepper, and garnish with fresh parsley before serving.

Per serving: Calories: 320 kcal; Fat: 15g; Carbs: 40g; Protein: 6g; Fiber: 5g; Sodium: 420mg

11 - Omelet with Bell Peppers and Goat Cheese

Preparation time: 10 min.

Cooking time: 10 min.

Servings: 2

Ingredients:

- 4 eggs
- 1 red bell pepper, cubed*
- 2 oz. goat cheese, crumbled
- Salt and pepper as required
- Fresh chives for garnish

Directions:

1. In your container, whisk the eggs then season with salt and pepper.

2. Heat a non-stick griddle over medium heat.

3. Include cubed bell pepper to the griddle then sauté until softened.

4. Pour the whisked eggs over the bell peppers then crumble goat cheese on top.

5. Cook until the eggs are set, then wrap the omelet in half.

6. Garnish with fresh chives and present.

Per serving: Calories: 320 kcal; Fat: 24g; Carbs: 6g; Protein: 20g; Fiber: 2g; Sodium: 300mg

12 - Spinach and Tomato Breakfast Quesadilla

Preparation time: 10 min.

Cooking time: 10 min.

Servings: 2

Ingredients:

- 4 gluten-free tortillas
- 1 cup fresh spinach
- 1 cup cherry tomatoes, carved*
- 1 cup lactose-free cheddar cheese, teared up
- Salt and pepper as required
- Olive oil for cooking

Directions:

1. Place a tortilla on a hot griddle lightly greased with oil over medium heat.

2. Layer with spinach, carved tomatoes, and teared up cheddar cheese.

3. Season with salt and pepper and top with another tortilla.

4. Cook until the cheese is dissolved and the tortilla is golden brown, then flip then cook the other side.

5. Repeat for the second quesadilla.

6. Slice and present warm.

Per serving: Calories: 380 kcal; Fat: 15g; Carbs: 45g; Protein: 15g; Fiber: 5g; Sodium: 480mg

13 - Peanut Butter Banana Toast

Preparation time: 5 min.

Cooking time: 0 min.

Servings: 2

Ingredients:

- 4 slices gluten-free bread
- 4 tbsps peanut butter
- 2 ripe bananas, carved
- Cinnamon for sprinkling (elective)

Directions:

1. Toast the gluten-free bread slices.

2. Place 1 tbsp of peanut butter on each slice.

3. Top with banana slices then sprinkle with cinnamon if desired.

4. Present instantly.

Per serving: Calories: 320 kcal; Fat: 15g; Carbs: 40g; Protein: 10g; Fiber: 6g; Sodium: 300mg

14 - Sweet Potato Hash with Poached Eggs

Preparation time: 15 min.

Cooking time: 20 min.

Servings: 2

Ingredients:

- 2 medium sweet potatoes, that is skinned and grated
- 1 tbsp olive oil
- 1 tsp paprika
- Salt and pepper as required
- 4 eggs
- Fresh parsley for garnish (elective)

Directions:

1. In your griddle, heat olive oil over medium heat.

2. Include grated sweet potatoes, paprika, salt, and pepper. Cook until sweet potatoes are soft and mildly crispy.

3. Meanwhile, poach the eggs in a separate pot of simmering water.

4. Present the sweet potato hash topped with poached eggs.

5. Garnish with fresh parsley if desired.

Per serving: Calories: 340 kcal; Fat: 15g; Carbs: 40g; Protein: 15g; Fiber: 6g; Sodium: 220mg

15 - Gluten-Free Buckwheat Waffles

Preparation time: 15 min.

Cooking time: 10 min.

Servings: 2 (4 waffles)

Ingredients:

- 1 cup buckwheat flour
- 1 tsp baking powder
- 1/2 tsp cinnamon
- 1 cup lactose-free almond milk
- 2 tbsps maple syrup
- 2 eggs
- 2 tbsps dissolved coconut oil
- Fresh blueberries for topping

Directions:

1. Warm up the waffle iron.

2. In your container, whisk collectively buckwheat flour, baking powder, and cinnamon.

3. In a distinct container, whisk collectively almond milk, maple syrup, eggs, and dissolved coconut oil.

4. Put wet components in to your dry components and mix until thoroughly blended.

5. Cook the batter in to your warmed up waffle iron as per to the manufacturer's guidelines.

6. Top with fresh blueberries and present.

Per serving: Calories: 400 kcal; Fat: 18g; Carbs: 50g; Protein: 10g; Fiber: 8g; Sodium: 180mg

16 - Avocado and Bacon Breakfast Sandwich

Preparation time: 15 min.

Cooking time: 10 min.

Servings: 2

Ingredients:

- 4 slices gluten-free bread
- 1 avocado, carved*
- 4 slices bacon, cooked
- 2 eggs, fried or scrambled
- Salt and pepper as required

Directions:

1. Toast the gluten-free bread slices.

2. On two slices of bread, layer carved avocado, bacon, and fried or scrambled eggs.

3. Season with salt and pepper.

4. Top using the rest of the slices of bread to make sandwiches.

5. Slice in half and present.

Per serving: Calories: 450 kcal; Fat: 25g; Carbs: 40g; Protein: 15g; Fiber: 8g; Sodium: 480mg

17 - Pineapple Mango Smoothie Bowl

Preparation time: 10 min.

Cooking time: 0 min.

Servings: 2

Ingredients:

- 2 cups frozen pineapple chunks
- 1 cup frozen mango chunks*
- 1 cup lactose-free yogurt
- 1/4 cup teared up coconut
- 2 tbsps chia seeds

Directions:

1. In a blender, blend frozen pineapple, frozen mango, and lactose-free yogurt.

2. Blend until smooth and creamy.

3. Pour the smoothie into two containers.

4. Top with teared up coconut and chia seeds.

5. Present instantly.

Per serving: Calories: 320 kcal; Fat: 12g; Carbs: 50g; Protein: 8g; Fiber: 10g; Sodium: 80mg

18 - Quiche with Spinach and Lactose-Free Cheese

Preparation time: 15 min.

Cooking time: 30 min.

Servings: 2

Ingredients:

- 4 eggs
- 1 cup lactose-free milk
- 1 cup fresh spinach, hand-torn
- 1 cup lactose-free cheese, teared up
- Salt and pepper as required
- Gluten-free pie crust

Directions:

1. Preheat the oven to 375°F.

2. In your container, whisk collectively eggs and lactose-free milk.

3. Stir in hand-torn spinach, teared up lactose-free cheese, salt, and pepper.

4. Pour the solution into a gluten-free pie crust.

5. Bake for 25-30 min. or until the quiche is set.

6. Allow it to cool mildly prior to slicing.

Per serving: Calories: 400 kcal; Fat: 25g; Carbs: 20g; Protein: 20g; Fiber: 2g; Sodium: 420mg

19 - Almond Flour Pancakes with Raspberry Compote

Preparation time: 15 min.

Cooking time: 10 min.

Servings: 2

Ingredients:

- 1 cup almond flour
- 2 eggs
- 1/2 cup lactose-free almond milk
- 1 tbsp maple syrup
- 1 tsp baking powder
- 1/2 tsp vanilla extract
- 1 cup fresh raspberries*
- 2 tbsps maple syrup (for compote)

Directions:

1. In your container, whisk collectively almond flour, eggs, almond milk, maple syrup, baking powder, and vanilla extract.

2. Heat a griddle over medium heat and lightly oil it.

3. Pour ¼ cup of batter onto your griddle for every pancake.

4. Cook the food until bubbles appear on the surface, then turn it over and continue cooking the other side.

5. In a saucepot, heat raspberries and 2 tbsps of maple syrup over low heat to make a compote.

6. Present pancakes with raspberry compote.

Per serving: Calories: 380 kcal; Fat: 25g; Carbs: 30g; Protein: 12g; Fiber: 8g; Sodium: 180mg

20 - Frittata with Sun-Dried Tomatoes and Basil

Preparation time: 15 min.

Cooking time: 20 min.

Servings: 2

Ingredients:

- 4 eggs
- 1/4 cup lactose-free milk
- 1/4 cup sun-dried tomatoes, chopped*
- 2 tbsps fresh basil, chopped
- Salt and pepper as required
- 1 tbsp olive oil

Directions:

1. Preheat the oven to 375°F.

2. In your container, whisk collectively eggs, lactose-free milk, chopped sun-dried tomatoes, chopped basil, salt, and pepper.

3. Heat olive oil in an oven-safe skillet at medium temperature.

4. Pour the egg solution in to your griddle then cook for 2-3 min. until the edges start to set.

5. Transfer the griddle to the warmed up oven then bake for 15-20 min. or until the frittata is fully cooked.

6. Allow it to cool mildly prior to slicing.

Per serving: Calories: 280 kcal; Fat: 20g; Carbs: 5g; Protein: 18g; Fiber: 1g; Sodium: 320mg

21 - Kiwi and Strawberry Breakfast Salad

Preparation time: 10 min.

Cooking time: 0 min.

Servings: 2

Ingredients:

- 2 kiwis, skinned and carved
- 1 cup strawberries, carved*
- 1 tbsp fresh mint, hand-torn
- 1 tbsp maple syrup (elective)
- 2 tbsps carved almonds

Directions:

1. In your container, blend kiwi slices, strawberry slices, and hand-torn mint.

2. Optional: Drizzle using maple syrup for sweetness.

3. Crumble carved almonds over the top.

4. Gently shake and present.

Per serving: Calories: 150 kcal; Fat: 6g; Carbs: 25g; Protein: 3g; Fiber: 7g; Sodium: 0mg

22 - Low FODMAP Breakfast Burrito

Preparation time: 15 min.

Cooking time: 10 min.

Servings: 2

Ingredients:

- 4 gluten-free tortillas
- 4 eggs, scrambled
- 1 cup spinach, hand-torn
- 1/2 cup tomatoes, cubed*
- 1/4 cup lactose-free feta cheese, crumbled
- Salt and pepper as required
- Salsa for presenting (elective)

Directions:

1. Warm the gluten-free tortillas as per to the package guidelines.

2. In your griddle, scramble the eggs over medium heat.

3. Assemble the burritos by placing scrambled eggs, hand-torn spinach, cubed tomatoes, and crumbled lactose-free feta on each tortilla.

4. Season with salt and pepper.

5. Wrap the sides of the tortillas then roll them up.

6. Optional: Present with salsa on the side.

Per serving: Calories: 350 kcal; Fat: 18g; Carbs: 30g; Protein: 18g; Fiber: 6g; Sodium: 720mg

23 - Coconut Flour Banana Muffins

Preparation time: 15 min.

Cooking time: 20 min.

Servings: 2 (6 muffins)

Ingredients:

- 1/2 cup coconut flour
- 1/2 tsp baking soda
- 1/4 tsp salt
- 3 ripe bananas, mashed
- 4 eggs
- 1/4 cup coconut oil, dissolved
- 1 tsp vanilla extract

Directions:

1. Warm up the oven to 350 deg. F then line a muffin tin using paper liners.

2. In your container, blend coconut flour, baking soda, and salt.

3. In a separate container, whisk collectively mashed bananas, eggs, dissolved coconut oil, and vanilla extract.

4. Put the wet components to the dry components and mix until thoroughly blended.

5. Split batter uniformly among your muffin cups.

6. Bake for 18-20 min. or until a toothpick that has been gently put into the middle comes out spotless.

7. Allow the muffins to cool thoroughly before serving.

Per serving: Calories: 350 kcal; Fat: 18g; Carbs: 40g; Protein: 10g; Fiber: 10g; Sodium: 320mg

24 - Rice Cake with Smoked Turkey and Tomato

Preparation time: 5 min.

Cooking time: 0 min.

Servings: 2

Ingredients:

- 4 rice cakes
- 8 slices smoked turkey
- 1 tomato, carved*
- Fresh basil leaves (elective)
- Salt and pepper as required

Directions:

1. Put the rice cakes on a plate or serving platter.

2. Layer each rice cake with 2 slices of smoked turkey and tomato slices.

3. Optional: Include fresh basil leaves for extra flavor.

4. Season with salt and pepper as required.

5. Present instantly.

Per serving: Calories: 200 kcal; Fat: 4g; Carbs: 30g; Protein: 12g; Fiber: 2g; Sodium: 480mg

25 - Maple Pecan Granola with Lactose-Free Yogurt

Preparation time: 10 min.

Cooking time: 20 min.

Servings: 2

Ingredients:

- 2 cups gluten-free oats
- 1/2 cup chopped pecans
- 1/4 cup maple syrup
- 2 tbsps coconut oil, dissolved
- 1 tsp vanilla extract
- 1 cup lactose-free yogurt
- Fresh blueberries for topping

Directions:

1. Warm up the oven to 325 deg. F afterward, prepare your baking sheet by lining it with parchment paper.

2. In your container, mix gluten-free oats, dissolved coconut oil, chopped pecans, maple syrup, and vanilla extract.

3. Spread the mixture evenly onto the prepared baking sheet.

4. Bake for 20 min., stirring halfway through.

5. Allow the granola to cool completely.

6. In serving containers, layer lactose-free yogurt with the maple pecan granola.

7. Top with fresh blueberries and present.

Per serving: Calories: 450 kcal; Fat: 24g; Carbs: 50g; Protein: 10g; Fiber: 8g; Sodium: 20mg

26 - Grilled Polenta with Blueberries

Preparation time: 15 min.

Cooking time: 10 min.

Servings: 2

Ingredients:

- 1 cup instant polenta
- 2 cups lactose-free almond milk
- 1 cup blueberries
- 1 tbsp maple syrup
- Sliced almonds for garnish (elective)

Directions:

1. In a saucepot, bring lactose-free almond milk to a simmer.

2. Slowly whisk in instant polenta and continue to whisk until thickened.

3. Pour the polenta into a square baking dish and allow it to relax and set.

4. Cut the polenta into squares and grill on a hot, mildly oiled pan for 2-3 min. on all sides.

5. In a separate pan, heat blueberries and maple syrup until the blueberries soften.

6. Present the grilled polenta topped with warm blueberries.

7. Optional: Garnish with carved almonds.

Per serving: Calories: 380 kcal; Fat: 8g; Carbs: 70g; Protein: 8g; Fiber: 6g; Sodium: 260mg

27 - Spinach and Feta Breakfast Wrap

Preparation time: 10 min.

Cooking time: 5 min.

Servings: 2

Ingredients:

- 4 gluten-free tortillas
- 2 cups fresh spinach
- 1/2 cup crumbled feta cheese
- 4 eggs, scrambled
- Salt and pepper as required
- Olive oil for cooking

Directions:

1. In your griddle, sauté fresh spinach in olive oil until wilted.

2. Inside the similar griddle, scramble the eggs then season with salt and pepper.

3. Lay out the gluten-free tortillas.

4. Split the sautéed spinach and scrambled eggs among the tortillas.

5. Crumble feta cheese on top.

6. Roll up the tortillas into wraps and present.

Per serving: Calories: 420 kcal; Fat: 18g; Carbs: 40g; Protein: 20g; Fiber: 4g; Sodium: 580mg

28 - Orange Ginger Turmeric Smoothie

Preparation time: 10 min.

Cooking time: 0 min.

Servings: 2

Ingredients:

- 1 cup lactose-free yogurt
- 1 orange, skinned and segmented
- 1/2 inch fresh ginger, that is skinned and grated
- 1/2 tsp ground turmeric
- 1 tbsp chia seeds
- Ice cubes (elective)

Directions:

1. In a blender, blend lactose-free yogurt, orange segments, grated ginger, ground turmeric, and chia seeds.

2. Blend until smooth.

3. If desired, include ice cubes and blend again.

4. Put into glasses and present instantly.

Per serving: Calories: 180 kcal; Fat: 6g; Carbs: 25g; Protein: 8g; Fiber: 6g; Sodium: 80mg

29 - Hash Browns with Bell Peppers and Eggs

Preparation time: 15 min.

Cooking time: 15 min.

Servings: 2

Ingredients:

- 2 potatoes, that is skinned and grated
- 1 green bell pepper, cubed
- 4 eggs
- 2 tbsps olive oil
- Salt and pepper as required
- Fresh chives for garnish

Directions:

1. Bring grated potatoes in a clean kitchen towel then squeeze out extra moisture.

2. In your container, blend grated potatoes, cubed bell pepper, salt, and pepper.

3. Heat olive oil on your griddle over medium heat.

4. Form potato solution into patties then cook until golden brown on all sides.

5. Inside the similar griddle, crack eggs then cook to desired doneness.

6. Present eggs over hash browns, garnish with fresh chives.

Per serving: Calories: 420 kcal; Fat: 24g; Carbs: 40g; Protein: 14g; Fiber: 5g; Sodium: 140mg

30 - Papaya and Lime Breakfast Boat

Preparation time: 10 min.

Cooking time: 0 min.

Servings: 2

Ingredients:

- 1 ripe papaya, divided and seeds taken out
- 1 lime, juiced
- 1 cup lactose-free yogurt
- 2 tbsps teared up coconut
- Fresh mint leaves for garnish

Directions:

1. Scoop out some of the papaya flesh to create a well in each half.

2. In your container, mix the scooped papaya with lime juice.

3. Fill each papaya half with lactose-free yogurt.

4. Top with the papaya-lime solution and teared up coconut.

5. Garnish with fresh mint leaves and present.

Per serving: Calories: 220 kcal; Fat: 10g; Carbs: 30g; Protein: 6g; Fiber: 5g; Sodium: 80mg

Lunch Recipes

31 - Turkey and Cranberry Lettuce Wraps

Preparation time: 15 min.

Cooking time: 0 min.

Servings: 2

Ingredients:

- 8 lettuce leaves (such as Bibb or Romaine)
- 1/2 lb. carved turkey breast
- 1/2 cup cranberry sauce (ensure it is free of high FODMAP components)*
- 1/4 cup pecans, chopped
- 1/4 cup feta cheese, crumbled (elective)

Directions:

1. Lay out the lettuce leaves on a clean surface.

2. Split the carved turkey among the lettuce leaves.

3. Spoon cranberry sauce over the turkey.

4. Crumble with chopped pecans and feta cheese.

5. Roll up the lettuce leaves, creating wraps.

6. Secure with toothpicks if needed and present.

Per serving: Calories: 320 kcal; Fat: 15g; Carbs: 30g; Protein: 20g; Fiber: 5g; Sodium: 480mg

32 - Quinoa and Grilled Chicken Bowl

Preparation time: 20 min.

Cooking time: 15 min.

Servings: 2

Ingredients:

- 1 cup cooked quinoa
- 1 lb. boneless, skinless chicken breasts, that is grilled and carved
- 1 cup cherry tomatoes, divided*
- 1 cup cucumber, cubed
- 1/4 cup fresh parsley, hand-torn
- 2 tbsps olive oil
- Salt and pepper as required
- Lemon wedges for presenting

Directions:

1. In your container, blend cooked quinoa, grilled chicken slices, cherry tomatoes, cucumber, and fresh parsley.

2. Mist using olive oil then shake to blend.

3. Season with salt and pepper as required.

4. Split the solution into two containers and present with lemon wedges.

Per serving: Calories: 420 kcal; Fat: 18g; Carbs: 30g; Protein: 35g; Fiber: 5g; Sodium: 120mg

33 - Tuna Salad with Cucumber and Olives

Preparation time: 10 min.

Cooking time: 0 min.

Servings: 2

Ingredients:

- 2 tins (5 oz each) tuna, drained
- 1 cucumber, cubed
- 1/4 cup Kalamata olives, carved
- 2 tbsps olive oil
- 1 tbsp lemon juice
- Fresh dill for garnish
- Salt and pepper as required

Directions:

1. In your container, blend drained tuna, cubed cucumber, and carved Kalamata olives.

2. Mist using olive oil and lemon juice, then shake to blend.

3. Season with salt and pepper as required.

4. Garnish with fresh dill and present.

Per serving: Calories: 300 kcal; Fat: 20g; Carbs: 5g; Protein: 25g; Fiber: 2g; Sodium: 480mg

34 - Grilled Shrimp and Vegetable Skewers

Preparation time: 20 min.

Cooking time: 10 min.

Servings: 2

Ingredients:

- 1/2 lb. shrimp, that is skinned and deveined
- 1 zucchini, carved into rounds*
- 1 green bell pepper, cut into chunks
- 1 tbsp olive oil
- 1 tsp paprika
- 1 tsp cumin
- Salt and pepper as required
- Lemon wedges for presenting

Directions:

1. Warm up the grill or grill pan.

2. In your container, shake shrimp, zucchini, and bell pepper with olive oil, paprika, cumin, salt, and pepper.

3. Thread shrimp and vegetables onto skewers.

4. Grill for 3-5 min. on all sides or until shrimp is fully cooked.

5. Present with lemon wedges.

Per serving: Calories: 280 kcal; Fat: 12g; Carbs: 10g; Protein: 30g; Fiber: 3g; Sodium: 320mg

35 - Eggplant and Tomato Stack

Preparation time: 15 min.

Cooking time: 20 min.

Servings: 2

Ingredients:

- 1 medium eggplant, carved into rounds*
- 2 tomatoes, carved**
- 1/2 cup lactose-free mozzarella cheese, teared up
- 1/4 cup fresh basil leaves
- 2 tbsps olive oil
- Salt and pepper as required
- Balsamic glaze for drizzling (elective)

Directions:

1. Preheat the oven to 375°F.

2. Place eggplant slices on your baking sheet and brush with olive oil.

3. Roast in the oven for 15-20 min. or until soft.

4. In your griddle, heat olive oil over medium heat.

5. Assemble stacks by layering eggplant rounds, tomato slices, and fresh basil leaves.

6. Crumble lactose-free mozzarella cheese between layers.

7. Repeat until you have two stacks.

8. Heat in your griddle until the cheese is dissolved.

9. Drizzle using balsamic glaze if desired and present.

Per serving: Calories: 280 kcal; Fat: 20g; Carbs: 20g; Protein: 8g; Fiber: 8g; Sodium: 160mg

36 - Lactose-Free Caprese Salad

Preparation time: 10 min.

Cooking time: 0 min.

Servings: 2

Ingredients:

- 2 cups cherry tomatoes, divided*
- 1 cup lactose-free mozzarella balls
- 1/4 cup fresh basil leaves
- 2 tbsps olive oil
- Salt and pepper as required
- Balsamic glaze for drizzling (elective)

Directions:

1. In your container, blend cherry tomatoes, lactose-free mozzarella balls, and fresh basil leaves.

2. Mist using olive oil then shake to blend.

3. Season with salt and pepper as required.

4. Drizzle using balsamic glaze if desired and present.

Per serving: Calories: 320 kcal; Fat: 26g; Carbs: 10g; Protein: 12g; Fiber: 2g; Sodium: 480mg

37 - Mediterranean Stuffed Bell Peppers

Preparation time: 20 min.

Cooking time: 25 min.

Servings: 2

Ingredients:

- 2 green bell peppers, seeds taken out
- 1 cup cooked quinoa
- 1/2 cup cucumber, cubed
- 1/4 cup Kalamata olives, carved
- 1/4 cup feta cheese, crumbled
- 2 tbsps fresh parsley, hand-torn
- 2 tbsps olive oil
- Salt and pepper as required
- Lemon wedges for presenting

Directions:

1. Preheat the oven to 375°F.

2. Place bell pepper halves in your baking dish.

3. In your container, blend cooked quinoa, cubed cucumber, carved Kalamata olives, crumbled feta cheese, hand-torn fresh parsley, olive oil, salt, and pepper.

4. Stuff each bell pepper half using the quinoa solution.

5. Bake for 25 min. or until the peppers are soft.

6. Present with lemon wedges.

Per serving: Calories: 350 kcal; Fat: 18g; Carbs: 35g; Protein: 10g; Fiber: 6g; Sodium: 325mg

38 - Salmon and Avocado Sushi Rolls

Preparation time: 30 min.

Cooking time: 0 min.

Servings: 2

Ingredients:

- 4 sheets nori seaweed
- 1 cup sushi rice, cooked then seasoned with rice vinegar
- 1/2 lb. fresh salmon, finely carved
- 1 avocado, carved*
- Soy sauce for dipping (ensure it's free of high FODMAP components)
- Pickled ginger for presenting (elective)
- Wasabi for presenting (elective)

Directions:

1. Put a sheet of nori on a bamboo sushi mat.

2. Disperse a thin layer of your sushi rice over the nori, leaving a mini border at the top.

3. Organize slices of fresh salmon and avocado along the bottom edge of the rice.

4. Carefully roll the sushi using the bamboo mat, sealing the edge with a little water.

5. Repeat with the rest of the nori sheets.

6. Slice each roll into bite-sized pieces.

7. Present with soy sauce, pickled ginger, and wasabi.

Per serving: Calories: 380 kcal; Fat: 18g; Carbs: 40g; Protein: 15g; Fiber: 5g; Sodium: 520mg

39 - Spinach and Feta Stuffed Chicken Breast

Preparation time: 20 min.

Cooking time: 25 min.

Servings: 2

Ingredients:

- 2 boneless, skinless chicken breasts
- 2 cups fresh spinach, hand-torn
- 1/2 cup feta cheese, crumbled
- 1 tbsp olive oil
- 1 tsp dried oregano
- Salt and pepper as required
- Toothpicks for securing

Directions:

1. Preheat the oven to 325°F.

2. In your griddle, heat olive oil over medium heat.

3. Include hand-torn spinach then sauté until wilted.

4. Take out from warm then stir in crumbled feta cheese.

5. Cut a pocket into each of your chicken breast then stuff with the spinach and feta solution.

6. Secure the openings with toothpicks.

7. Flavour your chicken breasts with dried oregano, salt, and pepper.

8. Bake for 25 min. or until chicken is fully cooked.

9. Take out toothpicks before serving.

Per serving: Calories: 320 kcal; Fat: 18g; Carbs: 4g; Protein: 35g; Fiber: 2g; Sodium: 420mg

40 - Lemon Herb Chicken Skewers

Preparation time: 15 min.

Cooking time: 15 min.

Servings: 2

Ingredients:

- 1 lb. boneless, skinless chicken thighs, that is cut into cubes
- 2 tbsps olive oil
- 1 tbsp fresh lemon juice
- 1 tsp dried thyme
- 1 tsp dried rosemary
- Salt and pepper as required
- Lemon wedges for presenting

Directions:

1. In your container, blend olive oil, fresh lemon juice, dried thyme, dried rosemary, salt, and pepper.

2. Include chicken cubes to the container and marinate for almost 15 min.

3. Warm up grill pan In a med-high temp.

4. Thread the marinated chicken onto skewers.

5. Grill the chicken skewers for around 6-8 min. on all sides or until fully cooked.

6. Present with lemon wedges.

Per serving: Calories: 380 kcal; Fat: 22g; Carbs: 2g; Protein: 40g; Fiber: 1g; Sodium: 180mg

41 - Zucchini Noodles with Pesto and Cherry Tomatoes

Preparation time: 15 min.

Cooking time: 5 min.

Servings: 2

Ingredients:

- 2 zucchini, spiralized into noodles*
- 1 cup cherry tomatoes, divided
- 1/4 cup pine nuts
- 1/2 cup fresh basil leaves
- 1/4 cup Parmesan cheese, grated
- 1/3 cup olive oil
- Salt and pepper as required

Directions:

1. In a blender, blend fresh basil, pine nuts, Parmesan cheese, salt, and pepper.

2. With your mixer on low speed, slowly drizzle in the olive oil until the pesto becomes smooth.

3. In a huge pan, sauté zucchini noodles for 3-5 min. until just soft.

4. Shake the zucchini noodles with cherry tomatoes and pesto.

5. Present instantly.

Per serving: Calories: 320 kcal; Fat: 30g; Carbs: 8g; Protein: 6g; Fiber: 3g; Sodium: 180mg

42 - Shrimp and Avocado Salad

Preparation time: 15 min.

Cooking time: 5 min.

Servings: 2

Ingredients:

- 1/2 lb. shrimp, that is skinned and deveined
- 2 cups mixed salad greens
- 1 avocado, carved*
- 1 cup cherry tomatoes, divided**
- 1/4 cup cucumber, carved
- 2 tbsps olive oil
- 1 tbsp fresh lemon juice
- Salt and pepper as required

Directions:

1. On your griddle, cook shrimp over medium heat until opaque, then fully cooked (about 2-3 minutes on all sides).

2. In a huge container, blend salad greens, carved avocado, cherry tomatoes, and cucumber.

3. Include cooked shrimp to the salad.

4. Mist using olive oil and fresh lemon juice.

5. Shake carefully to blend.

6. Season with salt and pepper as required.

7. Present instantly.

Per serving: Calories: 380 kcal; Fat: 28g; Carbs: 20g; Protein: 18g; Fiber: 8g; Sodium: 280mg

43 - Grilled Pork Chops with Pineapple Salsa

Preparation time: 15 min.

Cooking time: 15 min.

Servings: 2

Ingredients:

- 2 bone-in pork chops
- 1 cup pineapple, cubed
- 1/4 cup red bell pepper, cubed*
- 1 tbsp fresh cilantro, chopped
- 1 tbsp olive oil
- 1 tbsp lime juice
- Salt and pepper as required

Directions:

1. Warm up the grill or grill pan In a med-high temp.

2. Flavour pork chops with salt and pepper.

3. Grill pork chops for around 6-8 min. on all sides or until fully cooked.

4. In your container, blend cubed pineapple, cubed red bell pepper, chopped cilantro, olive oil, and lime juice.

5. Blend thoroughly to create the salsa.

6. Present grilled pork chops topped with pineapple salsa.

Per serving: Calories: 420 kcal; Fat: 26g; Carbs: 20g; Protein: 30g; Fiber: 3g; Sodium: 120mg

44 - Lactose-Free Margherita Pizza

Preparation time: 20 min.

Cooking time: 15 min.

Servings: 2

Ingredients:

- 2 gluten-free pizza crusts
- 1 cup lactose-free mozzarella cheese, teared up
- 1 cup cherry tomatoes, carved*
- 1/4 cup fresh basil leaves
- 2 tbsps olive oil
- Salt and pepper as required

Directions:

1. Warm up oven to a temp. specified on the pizza crust package.

2. Place pizza crusts on your baking sheet.

3. Evenly scatter torn lactose-free mozzarella over each crust.

4. Organize carved cherry tomatoes on top of the cheese.

5. Mist using olive oil then season with salt and pepper.

6. Bake according to the crust package guidelines until the cheese is dissolved then crust is golden.

7. Take out from the oven, top using fresh basil leaves, and present.

Per serving: Calories: 450 kcal; Fat: 20g; Carbs: 45g; Protein: 18g; Fiber: 4g; Sodium: 680mg

45 - Beef and Vegetable Lettuce Cups

Preparation time: 20 min.

Cooking time: 10 min.

Servings: 2

Ingredients:

- 1/2 lb. ground beef
- 1 cup carrots, julienned
- 1 cup zucchini, julienned*
- 1 cup green bell peppers, julienned
- 2 tbsps soy sauce (check for low FODMAP components)
- 1 tbsp sesame oil
- 1 tsp ginger, grated
- 1 tbsp green tops of green onions, chopped
- Bibb or iceberg lettuce leaves for presenting

Directions:

1. On your griddle, brown ground beef over medium heat.

2. Include julienned carrots, zucchini, and bell peppers to the griddle.

3. Stir in soy sauce, sesame oil, and grated ginger.

4. Cook until the vegetables are soft-crisp.

5. Stir in chopped green tops of green onions.

6. Spoon the beef and vegetable solution into lettuce leaves to create cups.

7. Present instantly.

Per serving: Calories: 380 kcal; Fat: 24g; Carbs: 20g; Protein: 24g; Fiber: 5g; Sodium: 820mg

46 - Teriyaki Tofu and Broccoli Stir-Fry

Preparation time: 15 min.

Cooking time: 15 min.

Servings: 2

Ingredients:

- 1 block firm tofu, pressed and cubed
- 2 cups broccoli florets
- 1 red bell pepper, carved*
- 2 tbsps low FODMAP teriyaki sauce
- 2 tbsps sesame oil
- 1 tbsp soy sauce (check for low FODMAP components)
- 1 tsp ginger, crushed
- 2 cups cooked jasmine rice

Directions:

1. In a huge griddle, warm sesame oil In a med-high temp.

2. Include cubed tofu then cook until golden brown on all sides.

3. Include broccoli florets, carved red bell pepper, and crushed ginger to the wok. Stir-fry until vegetables are soft-crisp.

4. Pour low FODMAP teriyaki sauce and soy sauce over the tofu and vegetables. Stir well to cover.

5. Present the stir-fry over cooked jasmine rice.

Per serving: Calories: 480 kcal; Fat: 20g; Carbs: 60g; Protein: 18g; Fiber: 8g; Sodium: 680mg

47 - Egg Salad Lettuce Wraps

Preparation time: 15 min.

Cooking time: 10 min.

Servings: 2

Ingredients:

- 4 hard-boiled eggs, chopped
- 1/4 cup mayonnaise (check for low FODMAP components)
- 1 tbsp Dijon mustard
- 1 tbsp chives, chopped
- Salt and pepper as required
- Bibb or iceberg lettuce leaves for wrapping
- Sliced tomatoes for garnish

Directions:

1. In your container, blend chopped hard-boiled eggs, mayonnaise, Dijon mustard, and chopped chives.

2. Blend thoroughly then season with salt and pepper as required.

3. Spoon the egg salad into lettuce leaves to create wraps.

4. Garnish with carved tomatoes and present.

Per serving: Calories: 350 kcal; Fat: 28g; Carbs: 4g; Protein: 16g; Fiber: 1g; Sodium: 420mg

48 - Quinoa Salad with Roasted Vegetables

Preparation time: 20 min.

Cooking time: 25 min.

Servings: 2

Ingredients:

- 1 cup quinoa, washed
- 2 cups mixed vegetables (e.g., zucchini, bell peppers, cherry tomatoes), chopped*
- 2 tbsps olive oil
- 1 tbsp balsamic vinegar
- Salt and pepper as required
- 1/4 cup fresh basil, hand-torn
- 1/4 cup pine nuts, toasted

Directions:

1. Preheat the oven to 400°F.

2. In your container, shake mixed vegetables with olive oil, balsamic vinegar, salt, and pepper.

3. Disperse the vegetables on your baking sheet and roast for 20-25 min. or until soft.

4. In a separate pot, cook quinoa using the package guidelines.

5. In a huge container, blend cooked quinoa with roasted vegetables.

6. Stir in fresh basil and top with toasted pine nuts.

7. Present warm or chilled.

Per serving: Calories: 450 kcal; Fat: 20g; Carbs: 55g; Protein: 12g; Fiber: 7g; Sodium: 20mg

49 - Lemony Chicken and Rice Bowl

Preparation time: 15 min.

Cooking time: 20 min.

Servings: 2

Ingredients:

- 1 lb. boneless, skinless chicken breasts, carved
- 1 cup jasmine rice, cooked
- 1 cup spinach, hand-torn
- 1 lemon, juiced
- 2 tbsps olive oil
- 1 tsp lemon zest
- Salt and pepper as required
- Fresh parsley for garnish

Directions:

1. In your griddle, warm olive oil In a med-high temp.

2. Include carved chicken then cook until browned then fully cooked.

3. In your container, blend cooked jasmine rice, hand-torn spinach, lemon juice, and lemon zest.

4. Stir in the cooked chicken.

5. Season with salt and pepper as required.

6. Garnish with fresh parsley and present.

Per serving: Calories: 420 kcal; Fat: 16g; Carbs: 40g; Protein: 30g; Fiber: 3g; Sodium: 120mg

50 - Grilled Vegetable and Polenta Stack

Preparation time: 20 min.

Cooking time: 15 min.

Servings: 2

Ingredients:

- 1 medium eggplant, carved
- 1 zucchini, carved*
- 1 red bell pepper, carved**
- 1 cup cherry tomatoes, divided
- 1 tube of pre-cooked polenta, carved
- 2 tbsps olive oil
- 1 tsp dried oregano
- Salt and pepper as required
- Fresh basil for garnish

Directions:

1. Warm up the grill pan In a med-high temp.

2. Brush eggplant, zucchini, red bell pepper, and polenta slices with olive oil.

3. Grill the vegetables and polenta slices for 3-5 min. on all sides or until grill marks appear.

4. Season with dried oregano, salt, and pepper.

5. Assemble the stack by layering grilled vegetables and polenta slices.

6. Garnish with fresh basil and present.

Per serving: Calories: 320 kcal; Fat: 18g; Carbs: 35g; Protein: 8g; Fiber: 9g; Sodium: 520mg

51 - Turkey and Cranberry Quinoa Stuffed Peppers

Preparation time: 20 min.

Cooking time: 25 min.

Servings: 2

Ingredients:

- 4 bell peppers, divided and seeds taken out
- 1/2 lb. ground turkey
- 1 cup cooked quinoa
- 1/4 cup cranberries (ensure they are free of high FODMAP components)*
- 1/4 cup green tops of green onions, chopped
- 1 tsp dried thyme
- Salt and pepper as required
- 1/2 cup lactose-free feta cheese, crumbled

Directions:

1. Preheat the oven to 375°F.

2. In your griddle, cook ground turkey until browned.

3. In your container, blend cooked ground turkey, cooked quinoa, cranberries, chopped green tops of green onions, dried thyme, salt, and pepper.

4. Stuff each bell pepper half with the turkey and quinoa solution.

5. Top with crumbled lactose-free feta cheese.

6. Bake for 25 min. or until the peppers are soft.

7. Present warm.

Per serving: Calories: 420 kcal; Fat: 18g; Carbs: 45g; Protein: 25g; Fiber: 7g; Sodium: 340mg

52 - Shrimp and Mango Lettuce Wraps

Preparation time: 20 min.

Cooking time: 5 min.

Servings: 2

Ingredients:

- 1/2 lb. shrimp, that is skinned and deveined
- 1 mango, skinned and cubed*
- 1/4 cup red bell pepper, cubed**
- 2 tbsps cilantro, chopped
- 1 tbsp lime juice
- 1 tbsp fish sauce
- 1 tsp sesame oil
- Bibb or iceberg lettuce leaves for wrapping

Directions:

1. In your griddle, cook shrimp over medium heat. until opaque then fully cooked (about 2-3 min. on all sides).

2. In your container, blend cooked shrimp, cubed mango, cubed red bell pepper, chopped cilantro, lime juice, fish sauce, and sesame oil.

3. Blend thoroughly to blend.

4. Spoon the shrimp and mango solution into lettuce leaves to create wraps.

5. Present instantly.

Per serving: Calories: 280 kcal; Fat: 6g; Carbs: 35g; Protein: 20g; Fiber: 5g; Sodium: 580mg

53 - Lactose-Free Greek Salad

Preparation time: 15 min.

Cooking time: 0 min.

Servings: 2

Ingredients:

- 2 cups mixed salad greens
- 1 cucumber, cubed
- 1 cup cherry tomatoes, divided*
- 1/2 cup Kalamata olives, carved
- 1/4 cup lactose-free feta cheese, crumbled
- 2 tbsps olive oil
- 1 tbsp red wine vinegar
- 1 tsp dried oregano
- Salt and pepper as required

Directions:

1. In a huge container, blend mixed salad greens, cubed cucumber, cherry tomatoes, carved Kalamata olives, and crumbled lactose-free feta cheese.

2. In a mini container, whisk collectively salt, olive oil, red wine vinegar, dried oregano, and pepper.

3. Spread the coating onto the salad and set it aside. then shake to blend.

4. Present instantly.

Per serving: Calories: 320 kcal; Fat: 26g; Carbs: 15g; Protein: 8g; Fiber: 5g; Sodium: 780mg

54 - Pesto Zoodle Bowl with Cherry Tomatoes

Preparation time: 15 min.

Cooking time: 5 min.

Servings: 2

Ingredients:

- 4 medium zucchinis, spiralized into zoodles*
- 1 cup cherry tomatoes, divided**
- 1/4 cup pine nuts, toasted
- 1/4 cup fresh basil leaves, hand-torn
- 2 tbsps olive oil
- 1 tbsp Parmesan cheese, grated
- Salt and pepper as required

Directions:

1. In a huge pan, sauté zucchini noodles in olive oil over medium heat. for 3-5 min. or until just soft.

2. Include cherry tomatoes then cook for an extra 2 min.

3. Stir in hand-torn fresh basil and toasted pine nuts.

4. Sprinkle with grated Parmesan cheese.

5. Season with salt and pepper as required.

6. Shake carefully and present.

Per serving: Calories: 280 kcal; Fat: 20g; Carbs: 18g; Protein: 8g; Fiber: 5g; Sodium: 160mg

55 - Turkey and Zucchini Burgers

Preparation time: 20 min.

Cooking time: 15 min.

Servings: 2

Ingredients:

- 1/2 lb. ground turkey
- 1 cup zucchini, grated then squeezed to take out extra moisture*
- 2 tbsps green tops of green onions, chopped
- 1 tsp garlic-infused olive oil
- 1 tsp dried oregano
- Salt and pepper as required
- Lettuce leaves for wrapping

Directions:

1. In your container, blend ground turkey, grated zucchini, chopped green tops of green onions, garlic-infused olive oil, dried oregano, salt, and pepper.

2. Mix until thoroughly blended.

3. Form the solution into burger patties.

4. Cook patties in your griddle In a med-high temp. for 6-8 min. on all sides or until fully cooked.

5. Present the turkey and zucchini burgers wrapped in lettuce leaves.

Per serving: Calories: 320 kcal; Fat: 16g; Carbs: 5g; Protein: 30g; Fiber: 2g; Sodium: 120mg

56 - Roasted Red Pepper & Goat Cheese Stuffed Chicken

Preparation time: 15 min.

Cooking time: 25 min.

Servings: 2

Ingredients:

- 2 boneless, skinless chicken breasts
- 1/4 cup roasted red peppers, chopped*
- 1/4 cup goat cheese, crumbled
- 1 tbsp olive oil
- 1 tsp dried thyme
- Salt and pepper as required

Directions:

1. Preheat the oven to 375°F.

2. Cut a pocket into each chicken breast.

3. In your container, mix chopped roasted red peppers, crumbled goat cheese, olive oil, dried thyme, salt, and pepper.

4. Stuff each chicken breast with the red pepper and goat cheese solution.

5. Flavour the outside of the chicken breasts using additional salt and pepper.

6. Bake for 25 min. or until chicken is fully cooked.

7. Present warm.

Per serving: Calories: 320 kcal; Fat: 18g; Carbs: 2g; Protein: 35g; Fiber: 1g; Sodium: 340mg

57 - Seared Tofu with Peanut Sauce

Preparation time: 15 min.

Cooking time: 10 min.

Servings: 2

Ingredients:

- 1 block firm tofu, pressed and carved
- 2 tbsps soy sauce (check for low FODMAP components)
- 1 tbsp peanut butter
- 1 tbsp sesame oil
- 1 tbsp rice vinegar
- 1 tsp maple syrup
- 1 tsp ginger, grated
- 1 tbsp green tops of green onions, chopped
- 1 tbsp sesame seeds for garnish

Directions:

1. In your container, whisk collectively soy sauce, peanut butter, sesame oil, rice vinegar, maple syrup, grated ginger, and chopped green tops of green onions.

2. Warm a non-stick griddle In a med-high temp.

3. Include carved tofu to the griddle and sear for 3-5 min. on all sides until golden brown.

4. Pour the peanut sauce over the tofu and let it simmer for 2 min.

5. Garnish with sesame seeds and present.

Per serving: Calories: 350 kcal; Fat: 24g; Carbs: 12g; Protein: 20g; Fiber: 3g; Sodium: 620mg

58 - Chicken and Quinoa Spring Rolls

Preparation time: 30 min.

Cooking time: 0 min.

Servings: 2

Ingredients:

- 4 rice paper sheets
- 1 cup cooked quinoa, cooled
- 1 cup cooked chicken breast, teared up
- 1 cup mixed salad greens
- 1/2 cucumber, julienned*
- 1/4 cup mint leaves
- 2 tbsps soy sauce (check for low FODMAP components)
- 1 tbsp sesame oil
- 1 tbsp rice vinegar
- 1 tsp maple syrup

Directions:

1. Pour warm water into a dish that is rather shallow.

2. Dip each rice paper sheet into water for 10-15 seconds until softened.

3. Lay softened rice paper on a clean surface.

4. Organize quinoa, teared up chicken, salad greens, cucumber, and mint leaves in the center of the rice paper.

5. In a mini container, whisk collectively soy sauce, sesame oil, rice vinegar, and maple syrup.

6. Drizzle the sauce over the fillings.

7. Wrap sides of your rice paper over the fillings then roll firmly.

8. Repeat for the rest of the sheets.

9. Slice each roll in half diagonally then present.

Per serving: Calories: 380 kcal; Fat: 10g; Carbs: 55g; Protein: 20g; Fiber: 6g; Sodium: 820mg

59 - Lemon Dill Salmon Patties

Preparation time: 20 min.

Cooking time: 10 min.

Servings: 2

Ingredients:

- 1 tin (14 oz.) tinned salmon, drained
- 1/2 cup gluten-free breadcrumbs
- 1 egg
- 2 tbsps lemon juice
- 1 tbsp fresh dill, chopped
- 1 tsp Dijon mustard
- 2 tbsps olive oil
- Lemon wedges for presenting

Directions:

1. In your container, blend tinned salmon, gluten-free breadcrumbs, egg, lemon juice, chopped fresh dill, and Dijon mustard.

2. Form the solution into patties.

3. In your griddle, heat olive oil over medium heat.

4. Cook salmon patties for 4-5 min. on all sides or until golden brown then fully cooked.

5. Present with lemon wedges.

Per serving: Calories: 320 kcal; Fat: 18g; Carbs: 20g; Protein: 22g; Fiber: 2g; Sodium: 720mg

60 - Vegetable and Rice Paper Rolls

Preparation time: 30 min.

Cooking time: 0 min.

Servings: 2

Ingredients:

- 8 rice paper sheets
- 1 cup cooked rice noodles, cooled
- 1 cup mixed vegetables (e.g., bell peppers, carrots, cucumber), julienned*
- 1/2 cup fresh basil leaves
- 1/4 cup peanuts, chopped
- 2 tbsps soy sauce (check for low FODMAP components)
- 1 tbsp rice vinegar
- 1 tsp maple syrup

Directions:

1. Pour warm water into a dish that is rather shallow.

2. Dip each rice paper sheet into water for 10-15 seconds until softened.

3. Lay softened rice paper on a clean surface.

4. Organize rice noodles, julienned vegetables, fresh basil, and chopped peanuts in the center of the rice paper.

5. In a mini container, whisk collectively soy sauce, rice vinegar, and maple syrup.

6. Pour the sauce over the fillings.

7. Wrap sides of the rice paper over the fillings then roll firmly.

8. Repeat for the rest of the sheets.

9. Slice each roll in half diagonally then present.

Per serving: Calories: 280 kcal; Fat: 10g; Carbs: 40g; Protein: 6g; Fiber: 4g; Sodium: 480mg

Dinner Recipes

61 - Lemon Herb Baked Chicken

Preparation time: 15 min.

Cooking time: 30 min.

Servings: 2

Ingredients:

- 2 boneless, skinless chicken breasts
- 2 tbsps olive oil
- 2 tbsps fresh lemon juice
- 1 tsp dried thyme
- 1 tsp dried rosemary
- Salt and pepper as required
- Lemon slices for garnish

Directions:

1. Preheat the oven to 400°F.

2. In your container, whisk collectively olive oil, lemon juice, dried thyme, dried rosemary, salt, and pepper.

3. Place chicken breasts in your baking dish and pour the lemon herb marinade over them.

4. Ensure the chicken is well covered using the marinade.

5. Bake for 25-30 min. or until the chicken is fully cooked.

6. Garnish with lemon slices and present.

Per serving: Calories: 320 kcal; Fat: 18g; Carbs: 2g; Protein: 35g; Fiber: 1g; Sodium: 160mg

62 - Beef and Broccoli Stir-Fry

Preparation time: 20 min.

Cooking time: 15 min.

Servings: 2

Ingredients:

- 1/2 lb. sirloin steak, finely carved
- 2 cups broccoli florets
- 1/4 cup soy sauce (check for low FODMAP components)
- 2 tbsps sesame oil
- 1 tbsp ginger, crushed
- 1 tbsp green tops of green onions, chopped
- 1 tbsp sesame seeds for garnish
- Cooked rice for presenting

Directions:

1. In a huge griddle, warm sesame oil In a med-high temp.

2. Include carved sirloin steak then cook until browned.

3. Include broccoli florets and crushed ginger to the wok. Stir-fry until the broccoli is soft-crisp.

4. Pour soy sauce over the beef and broccoli. Stir well to cover.

5. Sprinkle with chopped green tops of green onions and sesame seeds.

6. Present the stir-fry over cooked rice.

Per serving: Calories: 420 kcal; Fat: 25g; Carbs: 15g; Protein: 35g; Fiber: 4g; Sodium: 820mg

63 - Grilled Swordfish with Citrus Salsa

Preparation time: 15 min.

Cooking time: 10 min.

Servings: 2

Ingredients:

- 2 swordfish steaks
- 1 tbsp olive oil
- 1 tsp paprika
- Salt and pepper as required

Citrus Salsa:

- 1 orange, skinned and cubed
- 1 grapefruit, skinned and cubed
- 1 tbsp fresh cilantro, chopped
- 1 tbsp lime juice
- 1 tbsp olive oil
- Salt and pepper as required

Directions:

1. Warm up the grill or grill pan In a med-high temp.

2. Rub swordfish steaks with olive oil, paprika, salt, and pepper.

3. Grill swordfish for 4-5 min. on all sides or until fully cooked.

4. In your container, blend cubed orange, salt, cubed grapefruit, chopped cilantro, lime juice, olive oil, and pepper to create the citrus salsa.

5. Top grilled swordfish with citrus salsa and present.

Per serving: Calories: 380 kcal; Fat: 20g; Carbs: 18g; Protein: 30g; Fiber: 5g; Sodium: 280mg

64 - Ratatouille with Herbed Quinoa

Preparation time: 20 min.

Cooking time: 25 min.

Servings: 2

Ingredients:

- 1 zucchini, carved
- 1 eggplant, carved
- 1 red bell pepper, carved*
- 1 cup cherry tomatoes, divided*
- 2 tbsps olive oil
- 1 tsp dried thyme
- 1 tsp dried oregano
- Salt and pepper as required

Herbed Quinoa:

- 1 cup quinoa, washed
- 2 cups water or low FODMAP vegetable broth
- 1 tbsp fresh parsley, hand-torn
- 1 tbsp fresh chives, chopped

Directions:

1. Preheat the oven to 375°F.

2. In a baking dish, arrange carved zucchini, eggplant, red bell pepper, and cherry tomatoes.

3. Mist with olive oil then sprinkle with dried thyme, dried oregano, salt, and pepper.

4. Roast in the oven for 25 min. or until the vegetables are soft.

5. In a different pot, cook quinoa in water or low FODMAP vegetable broth as per to the package guidelines.

6. Fluff the cooked quinoa using a fork then stir in hand-torn fresh parsley and chives.

7. Present ratatouille over herbed quinoa.

Per serving: Calories: 420 kcal; Fat: 18g; Carbs: 60g; Protein: 10g; Fiber: 8g; Sodium: 40mg

65 - Lactose-Free Spinach and Feta Stuffed Portobello Mushrooms

Preparation time: 20 min.

Cooking time: 20 min.

Servings: 2

Ingredients:

- 4 portobello mushrooms, stems taken out
- 2 cups spinach, hand-torn
- 1/2 cup lactose-free feta cheese, crumbled
- 1 tbsp olive oil
- Salt and pepper as required
- Fresh parsley for garnish

Directions:

1. Preheat the oven to 375°F.

2. In your griddle, heat olive oil over medium heat.

3. Include hand-torn spinach to the griddle then cook until flaccid.

4. Take out from warm then stir in crumbled lactose-free feta cheese.

5. Place portobello mushrooms on your baking sheet.

6. Fill each mushroom with the spinach and feta solution.

7. Bake for 20 min. or until mushrooms are soft.

8. Garnish with fresh parsley and present.

Per serving: Calories: 280 kcal; Fat: 18g; Carbs: 15g; Protein: 12g; Fiber: 4g; Sodium: 480mg

66 - Pork and Pineapple Skewers

Preparation time: 15 min.

Cooking time: 10 min.

Servings: 2

Ingredients:

- 1/2 lb. pork tenderloin, that is cut into cubes
- 1 cup pineapple chunks
- 2 tbsps olive oil
- 1 tbsp soy sauce (check for low FODMAP components)
- 1 tsp ginger, grated
- 1 tsp maple syrup
- Salt and pepper as required

Directions:

1. In your container, whisk collectively olive oil, soy sauce, grated ginger, maple syrup, salt, and pepper.

2. Thread pork cubes and pineapple chunks alternately onto skewers.

3. Brush the skewers with the prepared marinade.

4. Grill the skewers In a med-high temp. for 5 min. on all sides or until the pork is fully cooked.

5. Present the pork and pineapple skewers.

Per serving: Calories: 320 kcal; Fat: 18g; Carbs: 20g; Protein: 22g; Fiber: 2g; Sodium: 720mg

67 - Shrimp Scampi with Zucchini Noodles

Preparation time: 20 min.

Cooking time: 10 min.

Servings: 2

Ingredients:

- 8 oz. shrimp, that is skinned and deveined
- 2 medium zucchinis, spiralized into noodles*
- 2 tbsps olive oil
- 1/4 tsp red pepper flakes*
- 1/4 cup white wine
- 1 tbsp lemon juice
- Salt and pepper as required
- Fresh parsley for garnish

Directions:

1. In your griddle, heat olive oil over medium heat.

2. Include red pepper flakes. Sauté until fragrant.

3. Include shrimp to the griddle then cook until pink and opaque.

4. Pour in white wine and lemon juice. Simmer for 2-3 min.

5. Include spiralized zucchini noodles to the griddle then shake until covered in the sauce.

6. Cook for an extra 2-3 min. until the zucchini noodles are just soft.

7. Season with salt and pepper as required.

8. Garnish with fresh parsley and present.

Per serving: Calories: 280 kcal; Fat: 14g; Carbs: 10g; Protein: 24g; Fiber: 3g; Sodium: 480mg

68 - Mediterranean Baked Cod

Preparation time: 15 min.

Cooking time: 20 min.

Servings: 2

Ingredients:

- 2 cod fillets
- 1 cup cherry tomatoes, divided
- 1/4 cup Kalamata olives, carved
- 2 tbsps olive oil
- 1 tbsp capers
- 1 tsp dried oregano
- Salt and pepper as required
- Lemon wedges for presenting

Directions:

1. Preheat the oven to 375°F.

2. Place cod fillets in your baking dish.

3. In your container, mix cherry tomatoes, carved Kalamata olives, olive oil, capers, dried oregano, salt, and pepper.

4. Spoon tomato and olive solution over the cod fillets.

5. Bake for 20 min. or until the cod is fully cooked.

6. Present with lemon wedges.

Per serving: Calories: 320 kcal; Fat: 18g; Carbs: 8g; Protein: 28g; Fiber: 2g; Sodium: 680mg

69 - Chicken and Vegetable Kebabs

Preparation time: 30 min. (includes marinating time)

Cooking time: 15 min.

Servings: 2

Ingredients:

• 1/2 lb. chicken breast, that is cut into cubes
• 1 zucchini, carved
• 1 red bell pepper, cut into chunks*
• 1 tbsp olive oil
• 1 tbsp soy sauce (check for low FODMAP components)
• 1 tbsp maple syrup
• 1 tsp Dijon mustard
• 1 tsp dried thyme
• Salt and pepper as required
• Wooden skewers, soaked in water

Directions:

1. In your container, whisk collectively olive oil, soy sauce, maple syrup, Dijon mustard, dried thyme, salt, and pepper.

2. Thread chicken cubes, zucchini slices, and bell pepper chunks onto the soaked wooden skewers.

3. Put the skewers in a shallow dish and brush with the marinade.

4. Let it marinate for almost 15 min.

5. Warm up the grill or grill pan In a med-high temp.

6. Grill the kebabs for 6-8 min., turning occasionally, until the chicken is fully cooked.

7. Present the kebabs warm.

Per serving: Calories: 320 kcal; Fat: 15g; Carbs: 20g; Protein: 25g; Fiber: 3g; Sodium: 620mg

70 - Eggplant Parmesan with Gluten-Free Breadcrumbs

Preparation time: 30 min.

Cooking time: 30 min.

Servings: 2

Ingredients:

• 1 eggplant, carved
• 1 cup gluten-free breadcrumbs
• 1/2 cup grated Parmesan cheese
• 2 eggs, whisked
• 2 cups low FODMAP marinara sauce
• 1 cup lactose-free mozzarella cheese, teared up
• Fresh basil for garnish
• Olive oil for drizzling

Directions:

1. Preheat the oven to 375°F.

2. Dip eggplant slices in whisked eggs and then coat with a solution of gluten-free breadcrumbs and grated Parmesan.

3. Put the covered eggplant slices on your baking sheet.

4. Bake for 20 min. or until the eggplant is golden brown.

5. In a baking dish, layer half of the marinara sauce, half of the baked eggplant slices, and half of the teared up lactose-free mozzarella.

6. Repeat the layers.

7. Mist with olive oil.

8. Bake for an extra 20-25 min. or until the cheese is dissolved and bubbly.

9. Garnish with fresh basil and present.

Per serving: Calories: 450 kcal; Fat: 22g; Carbs: 40g; Protein: 25g; Fiber: 8g; Sodium: 980mg

71 - Lemon Dill Salmon with Roasted Potatoes

Preparation time: 20 min.

Cooking time: 25 min.

Servings: 2

Ingredients:

- 2 salmon fillets
- 1 lemon, carved
- 2 tbsps olive oil
- 1 tbsp fresh dill, chopped
- 1 tsp Dijon mustard
- 1 tsp lemon zest
- Salt and pepper as required

Roasted Potatoes:

- 2 cups baby potatoes, divided
- 1 tbsp olive oil
- 1 tsp dried rosemary
- Salt and pepper as required

Directions:

1. Preheat the oven to 400°F.

2. In your container, whisk collectively olive oil, chopped fresh dill, Dijon mustard, lemon zest, salt, and pepper.

3. Put salmon fillets on your baking sheet covered using parchment paper.

4. Brush the salmon with the lemon dill solution and top with lemon slices.

5. In a separate container, shake divided baby potatoes with salt, olive oil, dried rosemary, and pepper.

6. Disperse the potatoes on the same baking sheet as the salmon.

7. Roast in the oven for 25 min. or until the salmon is fully cooked and the potatoes are golden brown.

8. Present the lemon dill salmon with roasted potatoes.

Per serving: Calories: 480 kcal; Fat: 28g; Carbs: 25g; Protein: 35g; Fiber: 4g; Sodium: 280mg

72 - Zoodle Carbonara with Bacon and Peas

Preparation time: 15 min.

Cooking time: 15 min.

Servings: 2

Ingredients:

- 2 medium zucchinis, spiralized into zoodles
- 4 slices bacon, diced
- 2 eggs
- 1/2 cup lactose-free Parmesan cheese, grated
- 1/2 cup frozen peas
- 2 tbsps olive oil
- Salt and pepper as required
- Fresh parsley for garnish

Directions:

1. In your griddle, cook diced bacon until crispy. Take out from the griddle and put away.

2. In your container, whisk collectively eggs and grated lactose-free Parmesan cheese.

3. In same griddle, include olive oil then sauté zucchini noodles until just soft.

4. Include frozen peas to the griddle then cook for 2 min.

5. Take out griddle from warm then quickly stir in the egg and cheese solution.

6. Put the cooked bacon back to the griddle then shake to blend.

7. Season with salt and pepper as required.

8. Garnish with fresh parsley and present.

Per serving: Calories: 350 kcal; Fat: 25g; Carbs: 12g; Protein: 18g; Fiber: 3g; Sodium: 580mg

73 - Teriyaki Chicken and Vegetable Skillet

Preparation time: 20 min.

Cooking time: 15 min.

Servings: 2

Ingredients:

- 1/2 lb. boneless, skinless chicken breasts, that is carved
- 2 cups mixed vegetables (bell peppers, zucchini, carrots), carved*
- 1/4 cup soy sauce (check for low FODMAP components)
- 2 tbsps maple syrup
- 1 tbsp sesame oil
- 1 tbsp ginger, crushed
- 1 tbsp green tops of green onions, chopped
- 1 tbsp sesame seeds for garnish
- Cooked rice for presenting

Directions:

1. In your container, whisk collectively soy sauce, maple syrup, sesame oil, crushed ginger, and chopped green tops of green onions.

2. Warm a big griddle In a med-high temp.

3. Include carved chicken to the griddle then cook until browned.

4. Include carved vegetables to the griddle then stir-fry until they are soft-crisp.

5. Pour teriyaki sauce over the chicken and vegetables. Stir well to cover.

6. Simmer for 2-3 min. until the sauce thickens.

7. Present over cooked rice then garnish with sesame seeds.

Per serving: Calories: 380 kcal; Fat: 15g; Carbs: 45g; Protein: 22g; Fiber: 4g; Sodium: 800mg

74 - Lactose-Free Margherita Risotto

Preparation time: 30 min.

Cooking time: 25 min.

Servings: 2

Ingredients:

- 1 cup Arborio rice
- 1/2 cup dry white wine
- 3 cups low FODMAP vegetable broth, heated
- 1 cup cherry tomatoes, divided*
- 1/4 cup lactose-free mozzarella cheese, teared up
- 2 tbsps lactose-free Parmesan cheese, grated
- 1 tbsp olive oil
- 1 tbsp fresh basil, hand-torn
- Salt and pepper as required

Directions:

1. In a huge pan, warm olive oil over medium heat.

2. Include Arborio rice then stir to cover with oil.

3. Pour in the white wine then cook until it's mostly evaporated.

4. Begin adding heated vegetable broth, one ladle at a time, mixing regularly until immersed.

5. Continue adding broth then stirring until the rice is creamy and al dente.

6. Stir in divided cherry tomatoes, teared up lactose-free mozzarella, and grated lactose-free Parmesan.

7. Season with salt and pepper as required.

8. Garnish with fresh basil and present.

Per serving: Calories: 450 kcal; Fat: 14g; Carbs: 65g; Protein: 8g; Fiber: 3g; Sodium: 750mg

75 - Maple Glazed Salmon with Roasted Brussels Sprouts

Preparation time: 20 min.

Cooking time: 25 min.

Servings: 2

Ingredients:

- 2 salmon fillets
- 2 tbsps maple syrup
- 1 tbsp Dijon mustard
- 1 tbsp olive oil
- 1 tsp soy sauce (check for low FODMAP components)
- 1 lb. Brussels sprouts, clipped and divided*
- Salt and pepper as required
- Lemon wedges for presenting

Directions:

1. Preheat the oven to 400°F.

2. In your container, whisk collectively maple syrup, Dijon mustard, olive oil, and soy sauce.

3. Place Brussels sprouts on your baking sheet then shake with half of the maple glaze.

4. Roast in the oven for 20 min.

5. Place salmon fillets on to your baking sheet and brush with the rest of the maple glaze.

6. Roast for an extra 15 min. or until the salmon is fully cooked.

7. Flavour Brussels sprouts and salmon with salt and pepper as required.

8. Present with lemon wedges.

Per serving: Calories: 420 kcal; Fat: 18g; Carbs: 30g; Protein: 30g; Fiber: 8g; Sodium: 340mg

76 - Baked Turkey Meatballs with Zucchini Noodles

Preparation time: 20 min.

Cooking time: 25 min.

Servings: 2

Ingredients:

- 1/2 lb. ground turkey
- 1/4 cup gluten-free breadcrumbs
- 1 egg
- 1/4 cup fresh parsley, hand-torn
- 1 tsp dried oregano
- Salt and pepper as required
- 2 medium zucchinis, spiralized into noodles*
- 1 cup low FODMAP marinara sauce
- Olive oil for drizzling
- Fresh basil for garnish

Directions:

1. Preheat the oven to 375°F.

2. In your container, blend ground turkey, gluten-free breadcrumbs, egg, chopped fresh parsley, dried oregano, salt, and pepper.

3. Shape the solution into meatballs then put them on your baking sheet.

4. Bake for 20-25 min. or until the meatballs are fully cooked.

5. In your griddle, heat low FODMAP marinara sauce over medium heat.

6. Include baked meatballs to the griddle then simmer for 5 min.

7. In a separate griddle, sauté zucchini noodles with olive oil until just soft.

8. Present the turkey meatballs over zucchini noodles.

9. Garnish with fresh basil.

Per serving: Calories: 320 kcal; Fat: 15g; Carbs: 20g; Protein: 25g; Fiber: 5g; Sodium: 680mg

77 - Pan-Seared Steak with Chimichurri Sauce

Preparation time: 15 min.

Cooking time: 10 min.

Servings: 2

Ingredients:

- 2 beef sirloin steaks
- Salt and pepper as required

Chimichurri Sauce:

- 1 cup fresh parsley, hand-torn
- 1/4 cup fresh cilantro, hand-torn
- 2 tbsps red wine vinegar
- 1/4 cup olive oil
- 1/4 tsp red pepper flakes
- Salt and pepper as required

Directions:

1. Flavour the steaks with salt and pepper.

2. In a hot griddle, sear the steaks for 3-4 min. on all sides for medium-rare or longer according to your preference.

3. Allow the steaks rest for a couple of min. prior to slicing.

4. In your container, blend chopped fresh parsley, chopped fresh cilantro, red wine vinegar, olive oil, red pepper flakes, salt, and pepper.

5. Present the carved steak drizzled with chimichurri sauce.

Per serving: Calories: 450 kcal; Fat: 30g; Carbs: 2g; Protein: 40g; Fiber: 1g; Sodium: 120mg

78 - Grilled Chicken Caesar Salad

Preparation time: 20 min.

Cooking time: 15 min.

Servings: 2

Ingredients:

- 2 boneless, skinless chicken breasts
- 1 tbsp olive oil
- Salt and pepper as required

Caesar Salad:

- 4 cups Romaine lettuce, hand-torn
- 1/4 cup lactose-free Parmesan cheese, shaved
- 1/4 cup gluten-free croutons
- Caesar dressing (check for low FODMAP components)

Directions:

1. Warm up the grill or grill pan In a med-high temp.

2. Brush chicken breasts using olive oil then season with salt and pepper.

3. Grill your chicken for 6-8 min. on all sides or until fully cooked.

4. Let chicken rest for a couple of min. prior to slicing.

5. In a huge container, blend chopped Romaine lettuce, shaved lactose-free Parmesan, and gluten-free croutons.

6. Include carved grilled chicken to the salad.

7. Drizzle using Caesar dressing then shake to blend.

8. Present the grilled chicken Caesar salad.

Per serving: Calories: 380 kcal; Fat: 20g; Carbs: 15g; Protein: 35g; Fiber: 3g; Sodium: 720mg

79 - Spaghetti Squash with Tomato Basil Sauce

Preparation time: 15 min.

Cooking time: 40 min.

Servings: 2

Ingredients:

• 1 medium spaghetti squash, that is divided and seeds taken out
• 2 tbsps olive oil
• Salt and pepper as required

Tomato Basil Sauce:

• 1 cup cherry tomatoes, divided*
• 1/4 cup fresh basil, chopped
• 2 tbsps olive oil
• Salt and pepper as required
• Lactose-free Parmesan cheese for garnish

Directions:

1. Preheat the oven to 400°F.

2. Brush the cut sides of spaghetti squash with olive oil then season with salt and pepper.

3. Put the squash, cut side down, on your baking sheet.

4. Roast in the oven for 30-40 min. or until the squash is fork-soft.

5. In your griddle, heat olive oil over medium heat.

6. Include divided cherry tomatoes then cook for 5 min.

7. Stir in chopped fresh basil then season with salt and pepper.

8. Use your fork to scrape the spaghetti squash into strands.

9. Top the spaghetti squash with tomato basil sauce and garnish with lactose-free Parmesan.

Per serving: Calories: 280 kcal; Fat: 18g; Carbs: 25g; Protein: 5g; Fiber: 5g; Sodium: 200mg

80 - Pesto Zucchini Noodles with Grilled Chicken

Preparation time: 20 min.

Cooking time: 15 min.

Servings: 2

Ingredients:

• 2 medium zucchinis, spiralized into noodles*
• 1/2 lb. boneless, skinless chicken breasts
• 2 tbsps pesto sauce
• 1 tbsp olive oil
• Salt and pepper as required
• Cherry tomatoes for garnish*
• Pine nuts for garnish

Directions:

1. Flavour the chicken breasts using salt and pepper.

2. Warm up the grill or grill pan In a med-high temp.

3. Grill the chicken for 6-8 min. on all sides or until fully cooked.

4. While your chicken is cooking, warm olive oil in your griddle over medium heat.

5. Put the zucchini noodles then sauté for 3-4 min. until just soft.

6. Shake the zucchini noodles with pesto sauce.

7. Slice the grilled chicken and present over the pesto zucchini noodles.

8. Garnish with cherry tomatoes and pine nuts.

Per serving: Calories: 380 kcal; Fat: 22g; Carbs: 10g; Protein: 35g; Fiber: 3g; Sodium: 480mg

81 - Stuffed Acorn Squash with Quinoa and Cranberries

Preparation time: 20 min.

Cooking time: 40 min.

Servings: 2

Ingredients:

- 1 acorn squash, divided and seeds taken out
- 1/2 cup quinoa, cooked
- 1/4 cup dried cranberries*
- 2 tbsps chopped pecans
- 1 tbsp olive oil
- 1 tbsp fresh parsley, chopped
- Salt and pepper as required

Directions:

1. Preheat the oven to 375°F.

2. Put the acorn squash halves on your baking sheet.

3. In your container, blend cooked quinoa, dried cranberries, chopped pecans, olive oil, chopped fresh parsley, salt, and pepper.

4. Fill each acorn squash half with the quinoa solution.

5. Bake for 35-40 min. or until the squash is fork-soft.

6. Present the filled acorn squash.

Per serving: Calories: 340 kcal; Fat: 15g; Carbs: 50g; Protein: 7g; Fiber: 7g; Sodium: 10mg

82 - Lactose-Free Margherita Zucchini Boats

Preparation time: 15 min.

Cooking time: 20 min.

Servings: 2

Ingredients:

- 2 zucchinis, divided lengthwise
- 1 cup cherry tomatoes, divided*
- 1/2 cup lactose-free mozzarella cheese, teared up
- 2 tbsps fresh basil, chopped
- 2 tbsps olive oil
- Salt and pepper as required

Directions:

1. Preheat the oven to 375°F.

2. Scoop out the center of each of your zucchini half to create a boat shape.

3. In your container, mix cherry tomatoes, lactose-free mozzarella cheese, chopped fresh basil, olive oil, salt, and pepper.

4. Fill each zucchini boat with the tomato and cheese solution.

5. Place zucchini boats on your baking sheet.

6. Bake for 15-20 min. or until the zucchini is soft.

7. Present the Margherita zucchini boats.

Per serving: Calories: 280 kcal; Fat: 20g; Carbs: 10g; Protein: 10g; Fiber: 3g; Sodium: 180mg

83 - Lemon Herb Grilled Shrimp

Preparation time: 15 min.

Cooking time: 5 min.

Servings: 2

Ingredients:

- 1/2 lb. shrimp, that is skinned and deveined
- 2 tbsps olive oil
- 1 tbsp fresh lemon juice
- 1 tsp fresh parsley, chopped
- 1 tsp fresh chives, chopped
- 1 tsp fresh thyme, chopped
- Salt and pepper as required
- Lemon wedges for presenting

Directions:

1. Warm up the grill or grill pan In a med-high temp.

2. In your container, mix shrimp with olive oil, fresh lemon juice, chopped fresh parsley, chopped fresh chives, chopped fresh thyme, salt, and pepper.

3. Thread shrimp onto skewers.

4. Grill shrimp for 2-3 min. on all sides or until they are opaque.

5. Take out shrimp from skewers and present with lemon wedges.

Per serving: Calories: 220 kcal; Fat: 15g; Carbs: 2g; Protein: 20g; Fiber: 0g; Sodium: 200mg

84 - Baked Cod with Lemon and Dill

Preparation time: 10 min.

Cooking time: 15 min.

Servings: 2

Ingredients:

- 2 cod fillets
- 1 lemon, carved
- 2 tbsps fresh dill, chopped
- 2 tbsps olive oil
- Salt and pepper as required

Directions:

1. Preheat the oven to 400°F.

2. Place cod fillets on your baking sheet covered using parchment paper.

3. Mist with olive oil over the cod fillets.

4. Sprinkle chopped fresh dill, salt, and pepper uniformly over the fillets.

5. Bring lemon slices on top of the cod.

6. Bake for 12-15 min. or until the cod is fully cooked then flakes simply using a fork.

7. Present the baked cod with lemon and dill.

Per serving: Calories: 250 kcal; Fat: 14g; Carbs: 2g; Protein: 28g; Fiber: 0g; Sodium: 300mg

85 - Seared Scallops with Garlic Butter

Preparation time: 10 min.

Cooking time: 5 min.

Servings: 2

Ingredients:

- 1/2 lb. scallops, patted dry
- 2 tbsps olive oil
- 2 tbsps unsalted lactose-free butter
- 1 tbsp fresh parsley, chopped
- Salt and pepper as required
- Lemon wedges for presenting

Directions:

1. Flavour scallops with salt and pepper.

2. In your griddle, warm olive oil In a med-high temp.

3. Include scallops to the griddle then sear for 2-3 min. on all sides or until they develop a golden crust.

4. Take out scallops from the griddle then put away.

5. Inside the similar griddle, dissolve lactose-free butter.

6. Sauté until fragrant.

7. Return the scallops to the griddle then shake in the garlic butter.

8. Sprinkle with chopped fresh parsley.

9. Present the seared scallops with lemon wedges.

Per serving: Calories: 280 kcal; Fat: 20g; Carbs: 6g; Protein: 18g; Fiber: 0g; Sodium: 350mg

86 - Roasted Vegetable and Quinoa Casserole

Preparation time: 20 min.

Cooking time: 30 min.

Servings: 2

Ingredients:

- 1 cup quinoa, cooked
- 1 zucchini, cubed*
- 1 red bell pepper, cubed*
- 1 cup cherry tomatoes, divided*
- 1 cup spinach, hand-torn
- 1/4 cup lactose-free Parmesan cheese, grated
- 2 tbsps olive oil
- 1 tsp dried oregano
- 1 tsp dried thyme
- Salt and pepper as required

Directions:

1. Preheat the oven to 400°F.

2. In a huge container, blend cubed zucchini, cubed red bell pepper, divided cherry tomatoes, hand-torn spinach, cooked quinoa, lactose-free Parmesan cheese, olive oil, dried oregano, dried thyme, salt, and pepper.

3. Transfer the solution to a baking dish.

4. Bake for 25-30 min. or until the vegetables are soft.

5. Present the roasted vegetable and quinoa casserole.

Per serving: Calories: 380 kcal; Fat: 18g; Carbs: 40g; Protein: 14g; Fiber: 7g; Sodium: 250mg

87 - Mediterranean Chicken Skillet

Preparation time: 15 min.

Cooking time: 20 min.

Servings: 2

Ingredients:

- 2 boneless, skinless chicken breasts
- 1 tbsp olive oil
- 1 tsp dried oregano
- 1 tsp dried thyme
- 1 tsp smoked paprika
- Salt and pepper as required
- 1 cup cherry tomatoes, divided*
- 1/2 cup Kalamata olives, that is eroded and carved
- 1/4 cup feta cheese, crumbled
- Fresh parsley for garnish

Directions:

1. Preheat the oven to 375°F.

2. In your container, mix olive oil, dried oregano, dried thyme, smoked paprika, salt, and pepper.

3. Rub the chicken breasts using the spice solution.

4. Warm an oven-safe griddle In a med-high temp.

5. Sear your chicken breasts for 2-3 min. on all sides.

6. Include divided cherry tomatoes and carved Kalamata olives to the griddle.

7. Transfer the griddle to the warmed up oven then bake for 15-20 min. or until the chicken is fully cooked.

8. Crumble feta over the top and garnish with fresh parsley.

9. Present the Mediterranean chicken griddle.

Per serving: Calories: 400 kcal; Fat: 20g; Carbs: 8g; Protein: 40g; Fiber: 2g; Sodium: 600mg

88 - Lemon Shrimp and Quinoa

Preparation time: 15 min.

Cooking time: 20 min.

Servings: 2

Ingredients:

- 1 cup quinoa, cooked
- 1/2 lb. shrimp, that is skinned and deveined
- 2 tbsps olive oil
- Zest of 1 lemon
- Juice of 1 lemon
- 1 tsp dried oregano
- Salt and pepper as required
- Fresh parsley for garnish

Directions:

1. In your griddle, warm olive oil In a med-high temp.

2. Place shrimp to the griddle then cook for 2-3 min. on all sides or until they are opaque.

3. Stir in cooked quinoa, lemon zest, lemon juice, dried oregano, salt, and pepper.

4. Shake everything together until thoroughly blended and fully heated.

5. Garnish with fresh parsley.

6. Present the lemon shrimp and quinoa.

Per serving: Calories: 400 kcal; Fat: 16g; Carbs: 45g; Protein: 25g; Fiber: 5g; Sodium: 400mg

89 - Zucchini and Tomato Gratin

Preparation time: 15 min.

Cooking time: 30 min.

Servings: 2

Ingredients:

- 2 zucchinis, finely carved
- 1 cup cherry tomatoes, divided*
- 1/4 cup lactose-free Parmesan cheese, grated
- 2 tbsps olive oil
- 1 tsp dried thyme
- Salt and pepper as required
- Fresh basil for garnish

Directions:

1. Preheat the oven to 375°F.

2. In your container, shake finely carved zucchinis and divided cherry tomatoes with olive oil, dried thyme, salt, and pepper.

3. Organize the zucchini and tomato solution in your baking dish.

4. Sprinkle grated lactose-free Parmesan cheese over the top.

5. Bake for 25-30 min. or until the vegetables are soft and the cheese is golden brown.

6. Garnish with fresh basil.

7. Present the zucchini and tomato gratin.

Per serving: Calories: 250 kcal; Fat: 18g; Carbs: 18g; Protein: 8g; Fiber: 4g; Sodium: 300mg

90 - Grilled Lamb Chops with Mint Chimichurri

Preparation time: 15 min.

Cooking time: 10 min.

Servings: 2

Ingredients:

- 4 lamb chops
- 2 tbsps olive oil
- 2 tbsps fresh mint, chopped
- 2 tbsps fresh parsley, chopped
- 1 tbsp red wine vinegar
- 1 tsp garlic-infused oil
- Salt and pepper as required

Directions:

1. Warm up the grill or grill pan In a med-high temp.

2. Brush lamb chops with olive oil then season with salt and pepper.

3. Grill your lamb chops for 4-5 min. on all sides for medium-rare or longer according to your preference.

4. In your container, mix chopped fresh mint, chopped fresh parsley, red wine vinegar, garlic-infused oil, salt, and pepper to create the chimichurri sauce.

5. Present grilled lamb chops drizzled with mint chimichurri.

Per serving: Calories: 500 kcal; Fat: 38g; Carbs: 1g; Protein: 38g; Fiber: 0g; Sodium: 120mg

Soups Recipes

91 - Carrot and Ginger Soup

Preparation time: 15 min.

Cooking time: 25 min.

Servings: 2

Ingredients:

- 1 lb. carrots, skinned and chopped
- 1 tbsp ginger, crushed
- 1 tbsp olive oil
- 4 cups low FODMAP vegetable broth
- Salt and pepper as required
- Fresh chives for garnish

Directions:

1. In a huge pot, heat olive oil over medium heat.

2. Include crushed ginger then sauté for 2 min. until fragrant.

3. Include chopped carrots to the pot then sauté for an extra 5 min.

4. Pour in low FODMAP vegetable broth and bring to a boil.

5. Reduce the heat then simmer for 15-20 min. or until the carrots are soft.

6. Use immersion mixer to puree soup until smooth.

7. Season with salt and pepper as required.

8. Garnish with fresh chives.

9. Present the carrot and ginger soup.

Per serving: Calories: 150 kcal; Fat: 7g; Carbs: 22g; Protein: 2g; Fiber: 5g; Sodium: 600mg

92 - Chicken and Rice Soup

Preparation time: 15 min.

Cooking time: 30 min.

Servings: 2

Ingredients:

- 1 tbsp olive oil
- 1/2 lb. boneless, skinless chicken thighs, that is cubed
- 1 carrot, skinned and carved
- 1 celery stalk, carved
- 1 cup cooked white rice
- 4 cups low FODMAP chicken broth
- 1 tsp dried thyme
- Salt and pepper as required
- Fresh parsley for garnish

Directions:

1. 1. In a huge pot, heat olive oil over medium heat.

2. Include cubed chicken then cook until browned.

3. Include carved carrot and celery to the pot then sauté for 5 min.

4. Pour in low FODMAP chicken broth and bring to a boil.

5. Include cooked white rice and dried thyme to the pot.

6. Simmer for 15-20 min. or until the chicken is fully cooked then the vegetables are soft.

7. Season with salt and pepper as required.

8. Garnish with fresh parsley.

9. Present the chicken and rice soup.

Per serving: Calories: 350 kcal; Fat: 12g; Carbs: 35g; Protein: 22g; Fiber: 2g; Sodium: 800mg

93 - Tomato Basil Soup with Lactose-Free Cream

Preparation time: 10 min.

Cooking time: 25 min.

Servings: 2

Ingredients:

- 1 tin (14 oz) crushed tomatoes*
- 1 cup low FODMAP chicken broth
- 1/2 cup lactose-free cream
- 2 tbsps olive oil
- 1 tsp dried basil
- Salt and pepper as required
- Fresh basil for garnish

Directions:

1. In your pot, blend crushed tomatoes, low FODMAP chicken broth, lactose-free cream, olive oil, and dried basil.

2. Simmer the solution over medium heat.

3. Simmer for 20 min., mixing irregularly.

4. Season with salt and pepper as required.

5. Use an immersion mixer to puree soup until smooth.

6. Garnish with fresh basil.

7. Present the tomato basil soup with lactose-free cream.

Per serving: Calories: 250 kcal; Fat: 20g; Carbs: 18g; Protein: 4g; Fiber: 4g; Sodium: 600mg

94 - Butternut Squash Soup

Preparation time: 20 min.

Cooking time: 30 min.

Servings: 2

Ingredients:

- 1 small butternut squash, that is skinned, sowed, and chopped*
- 1 tbsp olive oil
- 1/2 tsp ground cinnamon
- 1/4 tsp ground nutmeg
- 4 cups low FODMAP vegetable broth
- Salt and pepper as required
- Pumpkin seeds for garnish

Directions:

1. In your pot, heat olive oil over medium heat.

2. Include chopped butternut squash to the pot then sauté for 5 min.

3. Sprinkle ground cinnamon and ground nutmeg over the squash, then stir to cover.

4. Pour in low FODMAP vegetable broth and bring to a boil.

5. Reduce the heat then simmer for 20-25 min. or until the squash is soft.

6. Use immersion mixer to puree soup until smooth.

7. Season with salt and pepper as required.

8. Garnish with pumpkin seeds.

9. Present the butternut squash soup.

Per serving: Calories: 180 kcal; Fat: 8g; Carbs: 28g; Protein: 3g; Fiber: 5g; Sodium: 600mg

95 - Zucchini and Potato Soup

Preparation time: 15 min.

Cooking time: 25 min.

Servings: 2

Ingredients:

- 2 zucchinis, cubed*
- 2 potatoes, skinned and cubed
- 1 tbsp olive oil
- 4 cups low FODMAP vegetable broth
- 1 tsp dried thyme
- Salt and pepper as required
- Fresh chives for garnish

Directions:

1. In your pot, heat olive oil over medium heat.

2. Include cubed zucchinis and potatoes to the pot then sauté for 5 min.

3. Pour in low FODMAP vegetable broth and bring to a boil.

4. Include dried thyme, salt, and pepper to the pot.

5. Simmer for 15-20 min. or until the potatoes are soft.

6. Use immersion mixer to puree soup until smooth.

7. Season with additional salt and pepper if needed.

8. Garnish with fresh chives.

9. Present the zucchini and potato soup.

Per serving: Calories: 220 kcal; Fat: 5g; Carbs: 40g; Protein: 5g; Fiber: 5g; Sodium: 600mg

96 - Quinoa and Vegetable Minestrone

Preparation time: 15 min.

Cooking time: 30 min.

Servings: 2

Ingredients:

- 1/2 cup quinoa, washed
- 2 carrots, skinned and cubed
- 1 zucchini, cubed*
- 1 cup green beans, clipped and chopped
- 4 cups low FODMAP vegetable broth
- 1 tin (14 oz) cubed tomatoes*
- 1 tsp dried oregano
- 1 tsp dried basil
- Salt and pepper as required
- Fresh parsley for garnish

Directions:

1. In your pot, blend quinoa, cubed carrots, cubed zucchini, chopped green beans, low FODMAP vegetable broth, cubed tomatoes, dried oregano, dried basil, salt, and pepper.

2. Boil the solution In a med-high temp.

3. Reduce the heat then simmer for 20-25 min. or until the quinoa and vegetables are soft.

4. Season with additional salt and pepper if needed.

5. Garnish with fresh parsley.

6. Present the quinoa and vegetable minestrone.

Per serving: Calories: 320 kcal; Fat: 5g; Carbs: 60g; Protein: 12g; Fiber: 10g; Sodium: 700mg

97 - Spinach and Potato Soup

Preparation time: 15 min.

Cooking time: 25 min.

Servings: 2

Ingredients:

- 2 potatoes, skinned and cubed
- 2 cups baby spinach
- 1 tbsp olive oil
- 4 cups low FODMAP vegetable broth
- 1 tsp dried thyme
- Salt and pepper as required
- Lemon wedges for presenting

Directions:

1. In your pot, heat olive oil over medium heat.

2. Include cubed potatoes to the pot then sauté for 5 min.

3. Pour in low FODMAP vegetable broth and bring to a boil.

4. Include dried thyme, salt, and pepper to the pot.

5. Simmer for 15-20 min. or until the potatoes are soft.

6. Stir in baby spinach then cook until flaccid.

7. Season with additional salt and pepper if needed.

8. Present the spinach and potato soup with lemon wedges.

Per serving: Calories: 180 kcal; Fat: 5g; Carbs: 30g; Protein: 5g; Fiber: 5g; Sodium: 600mg

98 - Red Pepper and Tomato Soup

Preparation time: 15 min.

Cooking time: 30 min.

Servings: 2

Ingredients:

- 2 red bell peppers, cubed*
- 1 tin (14 oz) cubed tomatoes
- 1 tbsp olive oil
- 1 tsp dried basil
- 1 tsp dried oregano
- 4 cups low FODMAP vegetable broth
- Salt and pepper as required
- Fresh basil for garnish

Directions:

1. In your pot, heat olive oil over medium heat.

2. Include cubed red bell peppers to the pot then sauté for 5 min.

3. Include cubed tomatoes, dried basil, dried oregano, low FODMAP vegetable broth, salt, and pepper.

4. Boil the solution, then reduce the heat. then simmer for 20-25 min.

5. Use immersion mixer to puree soup until smooth.

6. Season with additional salt and pepper if needed.

7. Garnish with fresh basil.

8. Present the red pepper and tomato soup.

Per serving: Calories: 180 kcal; Fat: 7g; Carbs: 25g; Protein: 4g; Fiber: 6g; Sodium: 600mg

99 - Thai Coconut Shrimp Soup

Preparation time: 15 min.

Cooking time: 20 min.

Servings: 2

Ingredients:

- 1/2 lb. shrimp, that is skinned and deveined
- 1 tin (14 oz) coconut milk
- 2 cups low FODMAP chicken broth
- 1 red bell pepper, finely carved*
- 1 zucchini, julienned*
- 2 tbsps fish sauce
- 1 tbsp ginger, crushed
- 1 tbsp lime juice
- 1 tsp red curry paste
- Fresh cilantro for garnish

Directions:

1. In your pot, blend coconut milk, low FODMAP chicken broth, carved red bell pepper, julienned zucchini, fish sauce, crushed ginger, lime juice, and red curry paste.

2. Simmer the solution over medium heat.

3. Include shrimp to the pot then cook for 3-4 min. or until they are opaque.

4. Season with additional fish sauce or lime juice if needed.

5. Garnish with fresh cilantro.

6. Present the Thai coconut shrimp soup.

Per serving: Calories: 350 kcal; Fat: 20g; Carbs: 15g; Protein: 25g; Fiber: 3g; Sodium: 800mg

100 - Pumpkin and Turmeric Soup

Preparation time: 20 min.

Cooking time: 25 min.

Servings: 2

Ingredients:

- 1 tin (15 oz) pumpkin puree*
- 1 tbsp olive oil
- 1 tsp ground turmeric
- 1 tsp ground cumin
- 4 cups low FODMAP vegetable broth
- Salt and pepper as required
- Pumpkin seeds for garnish

Directions:

1. In your pot, heat olive oil over medium heat.

2. Include ground turmeric and ground cumin to the pot then sauté for 2 min.

3. Include pumpkin puree and low FODMAP vegetable broth to the pot.

4. Boil the solution, then reduce the heat. then simmer for 15-20 min.

5. Season with salt and pepper as required.

6. Use immersion mixer to puree soup until smooth.

7. Garnish with pumpkin seeds.

8. Present the pumpkin and turmeric soup.

Per serving: Calories: 220 kcal; Fat: 10g; Carbs: 30g; Protein: 5g; Fiber: 8g; Sodium: 600mg

101 - Lemon Chicken and Rice Soup

Preparation time: 15 min.

Cooking time: 30 min.

Servings: 2

Ingredients:

• 1/2 lb. boneless, skinless chicken thighs, that is cubed
• 1 carrot, skinned and carved
• 1 celery stalk, carved
• 1/2 cup cooked white rice
• 4 cups low FODMAP chicken broth
• 1 tbsp lemon zest
• 2 tbsps lemon juice
• 1 tsp dried thyme
• Salt and pepper as required
• Fresh parsley for garnish

Directions:

1. In your pot, blend cubed chicken, carved carrot, carved celery, cooked white rice, low FODMAP chicken broth, lemon zest, lemon juice, dried thyme, salt, and pepper.

2. Boil the solution In a med-high temp.

3. Reduce the heat then simmer for 20-25 min. or until the chicken is fully cooked and the vegetables are soft.

4. Season with additional salt and pepper if needed.

5. Garnish with fresh parsley.

6. Present the lemon chicken and rice soup.

Per serving: Calories: 300 kcal; Fat: 10g; Carbs: 30g; Protein: 20g; Fiber: 2g; Sodium: 800mg

102 - Roasted Eggplant Soup

Preparation time: 15 min.

Cooking time: 35 min.

Servings: 2

Ingredients:

• 1 eggplant, cubed
• 1 tbsp olive oil
• 1 tsp cumin
• 1 tsp smoked paprika
• 4 cups low FODMAP vegetable broth
• 1 cup cherry tomatoes, divided*
• Salt and pepper as required
• Fresh basil for garnish

Directions:

1. Preheat the oven to 400°F.

2. Shake cubed eggplant with olive oil, cumin, and smoked paprika.

3. Disperse the seasoned eggplant on your baking sheet and roast for 25-30 min. or until soft.

4. In your pot, bring low FODMAP vegetable broth to a simmer.

5. Include roasted eggplant and divided cherry tomatoes to the pot.

6. Simmer for 10 min.

7. Use immersion mixer to puree soup until smooth.

8. Season with salt and pepper as required.

9. Garnish with fresh basil.

10. Present the roasted eggplant soup.

Per serving: Calories: 180 kcal; Fat: 10g; Carbs: 20g; Protein: 4g; Fiber: 8g; Sodium: 600mg

103 - Lactose-Free Broccoli Cheddar Soup

Preparation time: 15 min.

Cooking time: 25 min.

Servings: 2

Ingredients:

- 2 cups broccoli florets
- 1 tbsp olive oil
- 2 cups lactose-free cheddar cheese, teared up
- 4 cups low FODMAP vegetable broth
- 1/2 cup lactose-free milk
- Salt and pepper as required
- Chives for garnish

Directions:

1. In your pot, heat olive oil over medium heat.

2. Include broccoli florets to the pot then sauté for 5 min.

3. Pour in low FODMAP vegetable broth and bring to a boil.

4. Reduce the heat then simmer for 15-20 min. or until the broccoli is soft.

5. Use immersion mixer to puree soup until smooth.

6. Stir in lactose-free cheddar cheese and lactose-free milk until the cheese is dissolved.

7. Season with salt and pepper as required.

8. Garnish with chives.

9. Present the lactose-free broccoli cheddar soup.

Per serving: Calories: 350 kcal; Fat: 20g; Carbs: 20g; Protein: 20g; Fiber: 6g; Sodium: 800mg

104 - Gazpacho with Cucumber and Bell Pepper

Preparation time: 15 min.

Cooking time: 0 min.

Servings: 2

Ingredients:

- 2 tomatoes, cubed*
- 1 cucumber, skinned and cubed*
- 1 red bell pepper, cubed
- 1/4 cup fresh parsley, chopped
- 1/4 cup olive oil
- 2 tbsps red wine vinegar
- 2 cups low FODMAP vegetable broth
- Salt and pepper as required
- Ice cubes (elective)
- Fresh basil for garnish

Directions:

1. In a blender, blend cubed tomatoes, cubed cucumber, cubed red bell pepper, chopped parsley, olive oil, and red wine vinegar.

2. Blend until smooth.

3. Transfer solution into a container then stir in low FODMAP vegetable broth.

4. Season with salt and pepper as required.

5. Cover and put in the fridge for almost 2 hrs before serving.

6. If desired, include ice cubes to individual containers before serving.

7. Garnish with fresh basil.

8. Present the gazpacho with cucumber and bell pepper.

Per serving: Calories: 200 kcal; Fat: 15g; Carbs: 15g; Protein: 3g; Fiber: 4g; Sodium: 600mg

105 - Potato Leek Soup

Preparation time: 15 min.

Cooking time: 30 min.

Servings: 2

Ingredients:

- 2 leeks, carved (use only the green parts)
- 2 tbsps olive oil
- 2 potatoes, skinned and cubed
- 4 cups low FODMAP vegetable broth
- 1 bay leaf
- Salt and pepper as required
- 1/4 cup lactose-free sour cream (elective)
- Chives for garnish

Directions:

1. In your pot, heat olive oil over medium heat.

2. Include carved leeks to the pot then sauté until softened.

3. Include cubed potatoes, low FODMAP vegetable broth, and a bay leaf to the pot.

4. Boil the solution, then reduce the heat. then simmer for 20-25 min. or until the potatoes are soft.

5. Take out the bay leaf and discard.

6. Use immersion mixer to puree soup until smooth.

7. Season with salt and pepper as required.

8. If desired, swirl in lactose-free sour cream.

9. Garnish with chives.

10. Present the potato leek soup.

Per serving: Calories: 250 kcal; Fat: 10g; Carbs: 35g; Protein: 4g; Fiber: 5g; Sodium: 700mg

Salads and Sides Recipes

106 - Cucumber and Tomato Salad with Feta

Preparation time: 10 min.

Cooking time: 0 min.

Servings: 2

Ingredients:

- 1 cucumber, carved
- 1 cup cherry tomatoes, divided*
- 1/4 cup lactose-free feta cheese, crumbled
- 2 tbsps olive oil
- 1 tbsp red wine vinegar
- Fresh oregano for garnish
- Salt and pepper as required

Directions:

1. In your container, blend carved cucumber and divided cherry tomatoes.

2. Place olive oil and red wine vinegar over your vegetables.

3. Shake the salad until well covered.

4. Crumble lactose-free feta cheese over the top.

5. Season with salt and pepper as required.

6. Garnish with fresh oregano.

7. Present the cucumber and tomato salad with feta.

Per serving: Calories: 150 kcal; Fat: 12g; Carbs: 8g; Protein: 4g; Fiber: 2g; Sodium: 300mg

107 - Roasted Brussels Sprouts with Bacon

Preparation time: 10 min.

Cooking time: 25 min.

Servings: 2

Ingredients:

- 2 cups Brussels sprouts, divided
- 2 slices bacon, cooked and crumbled
- 2 tbsps olive oil
- 1 tsp Dijon mustard
- Salt and pepper as required

Directions:

1. Preheat the oven to 400°F.

2. In your container, shake divided Brussels sprouts with olive oil, Dijon mustard, salt, and pepper.

3. Disperse Brussels sprouts on your baking sheet.

4. Roast for 20-25 min. or until golden brown and crispy.

5. Remove from the oven, then sprinkle crumbled bacon over the top.

6. Shake to blend.

7. Present the roasted Brussels sprouts with bacon.

Per serving: Calories: 200 kcal; Fat: 16g; Carbs: 10g; Protein: 6g; Fiber: 4g; Sodium: 300mg

108 - Quinoa and Roasted Vegetable Salad

Preparation time: 15 min.

Cooking time: 20 min.

Servings: 2

Ingredients:

- 1 cup quinoa, cooked
- 1 zucchini, cubed*
- 1 bell pepper, cubed
- 1 tbsp olive oil
- 1 tsp dried oregano
- Salt and pepper as required
- 1/4 cup pine nuts, toasted
- Fresh parsley for garnish

Directions:

1. In a pan, heat olive oil over medium heat.

2. Include cubed zucchini and cubed bell pepper to the pan.

3. Sprinkle dried oregano, salt, and pepper over the vegetables.

4. Sauté for 5-7 min. or until the vegetables are soft.

5. In your container, blend cooked quinoa and the sautéed vegetables.

6. Shake until well mixed.

7. Scatter toasted pine nuts over the top.

8. Garnish with fresh parsley.

9. Present the quinoa and roasted vegetable salad.

Per serving: Calories: 300 kcal; Fat: 14g; Carbs: 35g; Protein: 8g; Fiber: 5g; Sodium: 300mg

109 - Greek Salad with Lactose-Free Feta

Preparation time: 10 min.

Cooking time: 0 min.

Servings: 2

Ingredients:

- 2 cups mixed salad greens
- 1 cucumber, carved
- 1 cup cherry tomatoes, divided*
- 1/4 cup Kalamata olives, eroded
- 1/4 cup lactose-free feta cheese, crumbled
- 2 tbsps olive oil
- 1 tbsp red wine vinegar
- Fresh oregano for garnish
- Salt and pepper as required

Directions:

1. In a huge container, blend mixed salad greens, carved cucumber, divided cherry tomatoes, eroded Kalamata olives, and crumbled lactose-free feta cheese.

2. Place olive oil and red wine vinegar over the salad.

3. Shake until well covered.

4. Season with salt and pepper as required.

5. Garnish with fresh oregano.

6. Present the Greek salad with lactose-free feta.

Per serving: Calories: 250 kcal; Fat: 20g; Carbs: 15g; Protein: 6g; Fiber: 4g; Sodium: 500mg

110 - Grilled Asparagus with Lemon Zest

Preparation time: 10 min.

Cooking time: 10 min.

Servings: 2

Ingredients:

- 1 bunch asparagus, ends clipped*
- 2 tbsps olive oil
- Zest of 1 lemon
- Salt and pepper as required
- Lemon wedges for presenting

Directions:

1. Warm up a grill pan In a med-high temp.

2. Shake asparagus spears with olive oil, lemon zest, salt, and pepper.

3. Grill asparagus for 3-4 min. on all sides or until soft.

4. Transfer to a serving plate.

5. Mist using additional olive oil then garnish with extra lemon zest if desired.

6. Present the grilled asparagus with lemon zest.

7. Garnish with lemon wedges.

Per serving: Calories: 120 kcal; Fat: 10g; Carbs: 8g; Protein: 4g; Fiber: 4g; Sodium: 5mg

111 - Lactose-Free Coleslaw

Preparation time: 15 min.

Cooking time: 0 min.

Servings: 2

Ingredients:

- 2 cups teared up green cabbage
- 1 carrot, grated
- 1/4 cup lactose-free mayonnaise
- 1 tbsp Dijon mustard
- 1 tbsp apple cider vinegar
- 1 tsp maple syrup
- Salt and pepper as required
- Fresh chives for garnish

Directions:

1. In a huge container, blend teared up green cabbage and grated carrot.

2. In a mini container, whisk collectively lactose-free mayonnaise, salt, Dijon mustard, apple cider vinegar, maple syrup, and pepper.

3. Immediately place the dressing on top of the cabbage and carrot solution.

4. Shake until well covered.

5. Put in the fridge for a total of 30 min. before serving to let flavors meld.

6. Garnish with fresh chives.

7. Present the lactose-free coleslaw.

Per serving: Calories: 150 kcal; Fat: 10g; Carbs: 15g; Protein: 1g; Fiber: 4g; Sodium: 150mg

112 - Roasted Sweet Potato Wedges

Preparation time: 15 min.

Cooking time: 25 min.

Servings: 2

Ingredients:

- 2 medium sweet potatoes, cut into wedges
- 2 tbsps olive oil
- 1 tsp paprika
- 1 tsp cumin
- Salt and pepper as required
- Fresh parsley for garnish

Directions:

1. Preheat the oven to 400°F.

2. In your container, shake sweet potato wedges with olive oil, paprika, cumin, salt, and pepper.

3. Disperse the sweet potato wedges on your baking sheet in a single layer.

4. Roast for 20-25 min. or until golden brown and soft, flipping halfway through.

5. Transfer to a serving plate.

6. Garnish with fresh parsley.

7. Present the roasted sweet potato wedges.

Per serving: Calories: 200 kcal; Fat: 10g; Carbs: 25g; Protein: 2g; Fiber: 4g; Sodium: 70mg

113 - Quinoa Tabouleh

Preparation time: 15 min.

Cooking time: 15 min.

Servings: 2

Ingredients:

- 1 cup cooked quinoa, cooled
- 1 cup cucumber, finely cubed*
- 1 cup cherry tomatoes, divided*
- 1/4 cup fresh parsley, chopped
- 2 tbsps fresh mint, chopped
- 2 tbsps olive oil
- 1 tbsp lemon juice
- Salt and pepper as required
- Lemon wedges for presenting

Directions:

1. In your container, blend cooked quinoa, chopped fresh parsley, cubed cucumber, divided cherry tomatoes, and chopped fresh mint.

2. In a mini container, whisk collectively olive oil and lemon juice.

3. Immediately place the dressing on top of the quinoa solution then shake until thoroughly blended.

4. Season with salt and pepper as required.

5. Put in the fridge for almost 30 min. before serving.

6. Present the quinoa tabouleh with lemon wedges.

Per serving: Calories: 250 kcal; Fat: 14g; Carbs: 28g; Protein: 6g; Fiber: 5g; Sodium: 10mg

114 - Caprese Skewers with Balsamic Glaze

Preparation time: 15 min.

Cooking time: 0 min.

Servings: 2

Ingredients:

- 12 cherry tomatoes*
- 12 small fresh mozzarella balls
- Fresh basil leaves
- 2 tbsps balsamic glaze
- Salt and pepper as required

Directions:

1. Thread a cherry tomato, a fresh mozzarella ball, and a fresh basil leaf onto small skewers.

2. Organize the skewers on a serving plate.

3. Drizzle balsamic glaze over the skewers.

4. Season with salt and pepper as required.

5. Present the Caprese skewers with balsamic glaze.

Per serving: Calories: 200 kcal; Fat: 14g; Carbs: 10g; Protein: 8g; Fiber: 2g; Sodium: 300mg

115 - Lemon Roasted Broccoli

Preparation time: 10 min.

Cooking time: 20 min.

Servings: 2

Ingredients:

- 2 cups broccoli florets / heads
- 2 tbsps olive oil
- 1 tbsp lemon juice
- Salt and pepper as required
- Lemon wedges for presenting

Directions:

1. Preheat the oven to 400°F.

2. In your container, shake broccoli florets with salt, olive oil, lemon juice, and pepper.

3. Disperse the broccoli on your baking sheet.

4. Roast for 15-20 min. or until the broccoli is soft and mildly crispy.

5. Transfer to a serving plate.

6. Present the lemon roasted broccoli with lemon wedges.

Per serving: Calories: 150 kcal; Fat: 12g; Carbs: 10g; Protein: 4g; Fiber: 4g; Sodium: 50mg

116 - Potato Salad with Dijon Dressing

Preparation time: 15 min.

Cooking time: 15 min.

Servings: 2

Ingredients:

- 2 medium potatoes, boiled and cubed
- 1/4 cup green onions, carved
- 2 tbsps fresh parsley, chopped
- 2 tbsps Dijon mustard
- 2 tbsps olive oil
- 1 tbsp red wine vinegar
- Salt and pepper as required

Directions:

1. In your container, blend cubed boiled potatoes, carved green onions, and chopped fresh parsley.

2. In a mini container, whisk collectively salt, Dijon mustard, olive oil, red wine vinegar, and pepper.

3. Immediately place the dressing on top of the potato solution then shake until well covered.

4. Put in the fridge for 30 min. before serving.

5. Present the potato salad with Dijon dressing.

Per serving: Calories: 250 kcal; Fat: 12g; Carbs: 30g; Protein: 4g; Fiber: 4g; Sodium: 150mg

117 - Grilled Eggplant and Zucchini Salad

Preparation time: 15 min.

Cooking time: 10 min.

Servings: 2

Ingredients:

- 1 small eggplant, carved*
- 1 small zucchini, carved*
- 2 tbsps olive oil
- 1 tbsp balsamic vinegar*
- 1 tsp dried oregano
- Salt and pepper as required
- Fresh basil for garnish

Directions:

1. Warm up a grill pan In a med-high temp.

2. In your container, shake eggplant and zucchini slices with olive oil, balsamic vinegar, dried oregano, salt, and pepper.

3. Grill the slices for 4-5 min. on all sides or until soft and grill marks appear.

4. Organize the grilled eggplant and zucchini on a serving plate.

5. Garnish with fresh basil.

6. Present the grilled eggplant and zucchini salad.

Per serving: Calories: 180 kcal; Fat: 14g; Carbs: 12g; Protein: 2g; Fiber: 6g; Sodium: 10mg

118 - Lactose-Free Caesar Salad

Preparation time: 10 min.

Cooking time: 0 min.

Servings: 2

Ingredients:

- 4 cups romaine lettuce, chopped
- 1/4 cup lactose-free Caesar dressing
- 2 tbsps grated Parmesan cheese (elective)
- 1 cup cherry tomatoes, divided*
- Croutons (elective)

Directions:

1. In a huge container, shake chopped romaine lettuce with lactose-free Caesar dressing until well covered.

2. If using, sprinkle grated Parmesan cheese over the salad.

3. Include cherry tomatoes and croutons if desired.

4. Shake the salad until all components are uniformly dispersed.

5. Present the lactose-free Caesar salad.

Per serving: Calories: 150 kcal; Fat: 10g; Carbs: 12g; Protein: 4g; Fiber: 4g; Sodium: 250mg

119 - Spinach and Strawberry Salad with Almonds

Preparation time: 10 min.

Cooking time: 0 min.

Servings: 2

Ingredients:

- 4 cups baby spinach leaves
- 1 cup strawberries, hulled and carved*
- 1/4 cup carved almonds
- 2 tbsps olive oil
- 1 tbsp balsamic vinegar*
- Salt and pepper as required

Directions:

1. In a huge container, blend baby spinach leaves, carved strawberries, and carved almonds.

2. In a mini container, whisk collectively olive oil and balsamic vinegar.

3. Spread the coating onto the salad and set it aside. then shake until thoroughly blended.

4. Season with salt and pepper as required.

5. Present the spinach and strawberry salad with almonds.

Per serving: Calories: 180 kcal; Fat: 15g; Carbs: 10g; Protein: 4g; Fiber: 4g; Sodium: 20mg

120 - Mediterranean Quinoa Salad

Preparation time: 15 min.

Cooking time: 15 min.

Servings: 2

Ingredients:

- 1 cup cooked quinoa, cooled
- 1 cup cucumber, cubed*
- 1 cup cherry tomatoes, divided*
- 1/4 cup Kalamata olives, that is eroded and carved
- 2 tbsps feta cheese, crumbled
- 2 tbsps fresh parsley, chopped
- 2 tbsps olive oil
- 1 tbsp red wine vinegar
- Salt and pepper as required
- Lemon wedges for presenting

Directions:

1. In a huge container, blend cooked quinoa, cubed cucumber, divided cherry tomatoes, carved Kalamata olives, crumbled feta cheese, and chopped fresh parsley.

2. In a mini container, whisk collectively olive oil and red wine vinegar.

3. Immediately place the dressing on top of the quinoa solution then shake until thoroughly blended.

4. Season with salt and pepper as required.

5. Put in the fridge for almost 30 min. before serving.

6. Present the Mediterranean quinoa salad with lemon wedges.

Per serving: Calories: 300 kcal; Fat: 18g; Carbs: 30g; Protein: 8g; Fiber: 5g; Sodium: 300mg

Snacks and Desserts Recipes

121 - Almond and Pumpkin Seed Trail Mix

Preparation time: 5 min.

Cooking time: 0 min.

Servings: 2

Ingredients:

- 1/2 cup almonds
- 1/2 cup pumpkin seeds (pepitas)
- 1/4 cup sunflower seeds
- 1/4 cup dried cranberries*
- 1/4 tsp sea salt

Directions:

1. In your container, blend almonds, pumpkin seeds, sunflower seeds, and dried cranberries.

2. Season with sea salt then shake until well mixed.

3. Split the trail mix into two servings.

4. Present the almond and pumpkin seed trail mix.

Per serving: Calories: 250 kcal; Fat: 18g; Carbs: 20g; Protein: 8g; Fiber: 5g; Sodium: 150mg

122 - Dark Chocolate-Dipped Strawberries

Preparation time: 15 min.

Cooking time: 0 min.

Servings: 2

Ingredients:

- 1 cup strawberries, washed and dried*
- 1/4 cup 85% dark chocolate, dissolved

Directions:

1. Line a tray using parchment paper.

2. Dip each strawberry into the dissolved dark chocolate, coating about half of each strawberry.

3. Put the dipped strawberries on to your prepared tray.

4. Put in the fridge for 30 min. or until the chocolate hardens.

5. Present the dark chocolate-dipped strawberries.

Per serving: Calories: 120 kcal; Fat: 7g; Carbs: 15g; Protein: 2g; Fiber: 3g; Sodium: 0mg

123 - Lactose-Free Yogurt with Berries

Preparation time: 5 min.

Cooking time: 0 min.

Servings: 2

Ingredients:

- 1 cup lactose-free yogurt
- 1/2 cup blueberries
- 1/2 cup strawberries, carved*
- 1 tbsp maple syrup (elective)

Directions:

1. In two serving containers, divide the lactose-free yogurt.

2. Top with blueberries and carved strawberries.

3. If desired, drizzle with maple syrup.

4. Present the lactose-free yogurt with berries.

Per serving: Calories: 150 kcal; Fat: 3g; Carbs: 25g; Protein: 8g; Fiber: 3g; Sodium: 50mg

124 - Rice Cake with Peanut Butter and Banana

Preparation time: 5 min.

Cooking time: 0 min.

Servings: 2

Ingredients:

- 2 rice cakes
- 2 tbsps peanut butter (check for no added FODMAPs)
- 1 firm banana, carved

Directions:

1. Disperse 1 tbsp of your peanut butter on each rice cake.

2. Top with carved banana.

3. Present the rice cake with peanut butter and banana.

Per serving: Calories: 200 kcal; Fat: 9g; Carbs: 27g; Protein: 5g; Fiber: 3g; Sodium: 70mg

125 - Orange Slices with Tajin

Preparation time: 5 min.

Cooking time: 0 min.

Servings: 2

Ingredients:

- 2 oranges, skinned and carved*
- Tajin seasoning as required

Directions:

1. Organize orange slices on your serving plate.

2. Sprinkle Tajin seasoning over the orange slices to taste.

3. Present the orange slices with Tajin.

Per serving: Calories: 80 kcal; Fat: 0g; Carbs: 20g; Protein: 2g; Fiber: 4g; Sodium: 0mg

126 - Chocolate Avocado Mousse

Preparation time: 10 min.

Cooking time: 0 min.

Servings: 2

Ingredients:

- 1 ripe avocado*
- 3 tbsps unsweetened cocoa powder
- 3 tbsps maple syrup
- 1/2 tsp vanilla extract
- Tweak of salt
- Fresh blueberries for topping (elective)

Directions:

1. In a blender, blend the vanilla extract, ripe avocado, unsweetened cocoa powder, maple syrup, and a tweak of salt.

2. Blend until smooth and creamy.

3. Put in the fridge the chocolate avocado mousse for almost 1 hr.

4. Split into serving containers and top with fresh blueberries if desired.

5. Present the chocolate avocado mousse.

Per serving: Calories: 200 kcal; Fat: 12g; Carbs: 24g; Protein: 3g; Fiber: 7g; Sodium: 5mg

127 - Maple Cinnamon Roasted Nuts

Preparation time: 10 min.

Cooking time: 15 min.

Servings: 2

Ingredients:

- 1 cup mixed nuts (almonds, walnuts, pecans)
- 2 tbsps maple syrup
- 1 tsp ground cinnamon
- Tweak of salt

Directions:

1. Warm up the oven to 325 deg. F afterward, prepare your baking sheet by lining it with parchment paper.

2. In your container, shake the ground cinnamon, mixed nuts with maple syrup, and a tweak of salt.

3. Disperse the covered nuts on to your prepared baking sheet.

4. Bake for 12-15 min. or until the nuts are golden brown and fragrant.

5. Permit it to relax before serving.

6. Present the maple cinnamon roasted nuts.

Per serving: Calories: 250 kcal; Fat: 20g; Carbs: 15g; Protein: 6g; Fiber: 4g; Sodium: 50mg

128 - Grapes and Cheese Kabobs

Preparation time: 10 min.

Cooking time: 0 min.

Servings: 2

Ingredients:

- 1 cup grapes (choose green or red)*
- 1/2 cup firm lactose-free cheddar cheese, that is cut into cubes
- Wooden skewers

Directions:

1. Thread grapes and cheddar cheese cubes alternately onto the wooden skewers.

2. Repeat until each skewer is filled.

3. Present the grapes and cheese kabobs.

Per serving: Calories: 120 kcal; Fat: 6g; Carbs: 15g; Protein: 3g; Fiber: 2g; Sodium: 90mg

129 - Kiwi and Pineapple Fruit Salad

Preparation time: 10 min.

Cooking time: 0 min.

Servings: 2

Ingredients:

- 2 kiwis, skinned and carved
- 1 cup pineapple chunks*
- 1 tbsp fresh mint, chopped
- 1 tbsp maple syrup (elective)

Directions:

1. In your container, blend carved kiwis, pineapple chunks, and chopped fresh mint.

2. If desired, drizzle with maple syrup then shake carefully to blend.

3. Present the kiwi and pineapple fruit salad.

Per serving: Calories: 100 kcal; Fat: 1g; Carbs: 25g; Protein: 1g; Fiber: 4g; Sodium: 5mg

130 - Peanut Butter Energy Bites

Preparation time: 15 min.

Cooking time: 0 min.

Servings: 2

Ingredients:

- 1/2 cup rolled oats
- 1/4 cup peanut butter (check for no added FODMAPs)
- 2 tbsps maple syrup
- 1/4 cup teared up coconut (unsweetened)
- 1/4 cup dark chocolate chips

Directions:

1. In your container, blend rolled oats, peanut butter, maple syrup, teared up coconut, and dark chocolate chips.

2. Mix until thoroughly blended.

3. Put in the fridge the solution for 30 min.

4. Once chilled, roll into bite-sized balls.

5. Present the peanut butter energy bites.

Per serving: Calories: 200 kcal; Fat: 12g; Carbs: 20g; Protein: 5g; Fiber: 3g; Sodium: 40mg

131 - Lactose-Free Vanilla Pudding with Berries

Preparation time: 10 min.

Cooking time: 0 min.

Servings: 2

Ingredients:

• 1 cup lactose-free vanilla pudding (store-bought or homemade)
• 1 cup Low FODMAP mixed berries (eg. blueberries)*

Directions:

1. Split the lactose-free vanilla pudding into two serving containers.

2. Top every container with mixed berries.

3. Put in the fridge for 1 hr before serving.

4. Present the lactose-free vanilla pudding with berries.

Per serving: Calories: 180 kcal; Fat: 3g; Carbs: 35g; Protein: 2g; Fiber: 5g; Sodium: 120mg

132 - Popcorn with Olive Oil and Herbs

Preparation time: 10 min.

Cooking time: 5 min.

Servings: 2

Ingredients:

• 1/2 cup popcorn kernels
• 2 tbsps olive oil
• 1 tsp dried herbs (e.g., rosemary or thyme)
• Salt as required

Directions:

1. Pop the popcorn kernels using your preferred method.

2. In a mini saucepot, warm the olive oil and dried herbs over low heat for a couple of min. to infuse the flavors.

3. Drizzle the herbed olive oil over the popped popcorn, then toss to coat.

4. Season with salt as required.

5. Present the popcorn with olive oil and herbs.

Per serving: Calories: 150 kcal; Fat: 10g; Carbs: 15g; Protein: 2g; Fiber: 3g; Sodium: 150mg

133 - Rice Crackers with Smoked Salmon

Preparation time: 10 min.

Cooking time: 0 min.

Servings: 2

Ingredients:

• 20 rice crackers (check for no added FODMAPs)
• 4 oz smoked salmon, carved
• 1 tbsp chives, chopped
• Lemon wedges for presenting

Directions:

1. Organize the rice crackers on a serving plate.

2. Top each rice cracker with a slice of smoked salmon.

3. Chop chives over the smoked salmon.

4. Present the rice crackers with smoked salmon and lemon wedges.

Per serving: Calories: 200 kcal; Fat: 8g; Carbs: 24g; Protein: 10g; Fiber: 1g; Sodium: 500mg

134 - Dark Chocolate Almond Clusters

Preparation time: 15 min.

Cooking time: 0 min.

Servings: 2

Ingredients:

• 1/2 cup dark chocolate chips
• 1/2 cup almonds
• Sea salt as required

Directions:

1. In your heatproof container, dissolve the dark chocolate chips using a microwave or double boiler.

2. Stir in the almonds until well covered with chocolate.

3. Drop spoonfuls of the chocolate-covered almonds onto a parchment-covered tray.

4. Season with sea salt as required.

5. Put in the fridge for 30 min. or until the chocolate is set.

6. Present the dark chocolate almond clusters.

Per serving: Calories: 250 kcal; Fat: 18g; Carbs: 15g; Protein: 5g; Fiber: 3g; Sodium: 5mg

135 - Mango and Lime Sorbet

Preparation time: 10 min.

Cooking time: 0 min.

Servings: 2

Ingredients:

- 2 cups frozen mango chunks*
- Juice of 1 lime
- 2 tbsps maple syrup (elective)

Directions:

1. In your mixer, blend the frozen mango chunks, lime juice, and maple syrup (if using).

2. Blend until smooth.

3. If the sorbet is too dense, you can add a small amount of water to achieve the desired consistency.

4. Transfer the solution to a freezer-safe container then freeze for almost 4 hrs.

5. Before serving, let your sorbet sit at room temp. for a couple of min. to soften.

6. Present the mango and lime sorbet.

Per serving: Calories: 150 kcal; Fat: 0g; Carbs: 40g; Protein: 1g; Fiber: 3g; Sodium: 0mg

136 - Lactose-Free Ice Cream with Chocolate Sauce

Preparation time: 10 min.

Cooking time: 0 min.

Servings: 2

Ingredients:

- 2 cups lactose-free vanilla ice cream
- 1/4 cup dark chocolate, dissolved
- 1 tbsp chopped nuts (elective)

Directions:

1. Scoop the lactose-free vanilla ice cream into serving containers.

2. Drizzle melted dark chocolate over the ice cream.

3. Garnish with chopped nuts if desired.

4. Freeze for an extra 10-15 min. for the chocolate to set.

5. Present the lactose-free ice cream with chocolate sauce.

Per serving: Calories: 250 kcal; Fat: 15g; Carbs: 30g; Protein: 4g; Fiber: 2g; Sodium: 60mg

137 - Greek Yogurt with Honey and Walnuts

Preparation time: 5 min.

Cooking time: 0 min.

Servings: 2

Ingredients:

- 2 cups lactose-free Greek yogurt
- 2 tbsps honey*
- 2 tbsps chopped walnuts

Directions:

1. Split the lactose-free Greek yogurt into two serving containers.

2. Drizzle 1 tbsp of honey into each container.

3. Scatter chopped walnuts over the yogurt.

4. Present the Greek yogurt using honey and walnuts.

Per serving: Calories: 250 kcal; Fat: 10g; Carbs: 30g; Protein: 14g; Fiber: 1g; Sodium: 80mg

138 - Strawberry and Kiwi Popsicles

Preparation time: 10 min.

Cooking time: 0 min.

Servings: 2

Ingredients:

- 1 cup strawberries, hulled and carved*
- 1 kiwi, skinned and carved
- 1 cup lactose-free yogurt
- 2 tbsps maple syrup (elective)

Directions:

1. In a blender, blend the strawberries, kiwi, lactose-free yogurt, and maple syrup (if using).

2. Blend until smooth.

3. Pour the solution into popsicle molds.

4. Place popsicle sticks then freeze for almost 4 hrs.

5. Before serving, run the molds under warm water to release the popsicles.

6. Present the strawberry and kiwi popsicles.

Per serving: Calories: 120 kcal; Fat: 3g; Carbs: 22g; Protein: 4g; Fiber: 3g; Sodium: 40mg

139 - Nut and Seed Bars

Preparation time: 15 min.

Cooking time: 0 min.

Servings: 2

Ingredients:

- 1/2 cup mixed nuts (almonds, walnuts, or other low FODMAP nuts)
- 1/4 cup mixed seeds (sunflower seeds, pumpkin seeds)
- 2 tbsps chia seeds
- 2 tbsps teared up coconut (unsweetened)
- 1/4 cup maple syrup
- 2 tbsps coconut oil, dissolved
- 1/2 tsp vanilla extract
- Tweak of salt

Directions:

1. In your blending container, pulse the mixed nuts and seeds until coarsely chopped.

2. In your container, blend the chopped nuts and seeds with chia seeds, dissolved coconut oil, vanilla extract, teared up coconut, maple syrup, and a tweak of salt.

3. Press solution into a covered pan and put in the fridge for almost 1 hr.

4. Once set, cut into bars.

5. Present the nut and seed bars.

Per serving: Calories: 300 kcal; Fat: 24g; Carbs: 18g; Protein: 6g; Fiber: 5g; Sodium: 50mg

140 - Roasted Chickpeas with Paprika

Preparation time: 10 min.

Cooking time: 25 min.

Servings: 2

Ingredients:

- 1 tin (15 oz) chickpeas, that is drained and washed
- 1 tbsp olive oil
- 1 tsp paprika
- 1/2 tsp cumin
- 1/4 tsp cayenne pepper
- Salt as required

Directions:

1. Warm up the oven to 400 deg. F afterward, prepare your baking sheet by lining it with parchment paper.

2. Pat your chickpeas dry using a paper towel.

3. In your container, shake the chickpeas with olive oil, paprika, cumin, cayenne pepper, and salt.

4. Disperse the chickpeas on to your prepared baking sheet.

5. Roast for 25 min. or until crispy, shaking the pan occasionally.

6. Permit it to relax before serving.

7. Present the roasted chickpeas with paprika.

Per serving: Calories: 200 kcal; Fat: 7g; Carbs: 27g; Protein: 8g; Fiber: 6g; Sodium: 300mg

141 - Pineapple Coconut Chia Pudding

Preparation time: 10 min.

Cooking time: 0 min.

Servings: 2

Ingredients:

- 1 cup lactose-free coconut milk
- 1/4 cup chia seeds
- 1/2 cup pineapple chunks*
- 2 tbsps teared up coconut (unsweetened)
- 1 tbsp maple syrup (elective)

Directions:

1. In your container, whisk collectively coconut milk and chia seeds.

2. Allow it to relax for 10 min., whisking occasionally to avoid clumps.

3. Stir in pineapple chunks, teared up coconut, and maple syrup (if using).

4. Put in the fridge for almost 4 hrs or overnight.

5. Stir before serving.

6. Present the pineapple coconut chia pudding.

Per serving: Calories: 220 kcal; Fat: 13g; Carbs: 22g; Protein: 4g; Fiber: 10g; Sodium: 20mg

142 - Lemon Sorbet with Mint

Preparation time: 10 min.

Cooking time: 0 min.

Servings: 2

Ingredients:

- 1 cup water
- 1/2 cup sugar
- Zest of 1 lemon
- 1/2 cup fresh lemon juice
- 1 tbsp fresh mint, chopped

Directions:

1. In a saucepot, heat water, sugar, and lemon zest over medium heat., stirring until the sugar dissolves.

2. Take out from warm and allow it to relax.

3. Stir in fresh lemon juice and chopped mint.

4. Place solution into an ice cream maker then churn as per to the manufacturer's guidelines.

5. PLace to a freezer-safe container and freeze for almost 4 hrs.

6. Allow to soften at room temp. for a couple of min. before serving.

7. Present the lemon sorbet with mint.

Per serving: Calories: 150 kcal; Fat: 0g; Carbs: 40g; Protein: 0g; Fiber: 1g; Sodium: 5mg

143 - Rice Cake with Avocado and Cherry Tomatoes

Preparation time: 5 min.

Cooking time: 0 min.

Servings: 2

Ingredients:

- 2 rice cakes
- 1 ripe avocado, carved*
- 1 cup cherry tomatoes, divided*
- Salt and pepper as required
- Fresh basil leaves for garnish

Directions:

1. Put the rice cakes on your serving plate.

2. Top each rice cake with carved avocado and divided cherry tomatoes.

3. Season with salt and pepper as required.

4. Garnish with fresh basil leaves.

5. Present the rice cake with avocado and cherry tomatoes.

Per serving: Calories: 200 kcal; Fat: 12g; Carbs: 20g; Protein: 3g; Fiber: 6g; Sodium: 150mg

144 - Blueberry Almond Granola Bars

Preparation time: 15 min.

Cooking time: 0 min.

Servings: 2

Ingredients:

- 1 cup oats (ensure they are gluten-free)
- 1/2 cup almond butter
- 1/4 cup maple syrup
- 1/4 cup blueberries
- 1/4 cup carved almonds
- Tweak of salt

Directions:

1. In your container, blend oats, almond butter, maple syrup, blueberries, carved almonds, and a tweak of salt.

2. Mix until thoroughly blended.

3. Press solution into a covered pan then put in the fridge for almost 1 hr.

4. Once set, cut into granola bars.

5. Present the blueberry almond granola bars.

Per serving: Calories: 350 kcal; Fat: 20g; Carbs: 35g; Protein: 8g; Fiber: 6g; Sodium: 50mg

145 - Chocolate Banana Smoothie

Preparation time: 5 min.

Cooking time: 0 min.

Servings: 2

Ingredients:

- 2 medium ripe bananas
- 2 cups lactose-free almond milk
- 2 tbsps unsweetened cocoa powder
- 1 tbsp maple syrup
- Ice cubes (elective)

Directions:

1. In a blender, blend ripe bananas, lactose-free almond milk, cocoa powder, and maple syrup.

2. Blend until smooth.

3. Include ice cubes if desired then blend again.

4. Put into glasses and present the chocolate banana smoothie.

Per serving: Calories: 180 kcal; Fat: 4g; Carbs: 40g; Protein: 3g; Fiber: 7g; Sodium: 200mg

146 - Lactose-Free Cheesecake Bites

Preparation time: 15 min.

Cooking time: 0 min.

Servings: 2

Ingredients:

- 1 cup lactose-free cream cheese
- 2 tbsps maple syrup
- 1 tsp vanilla extract
- Fresh berries for topping (elective)

Directions:

1. In your container, beat together lactose-free cream cheese, maple syrup, and vanilla extract until smooth.

2. Spoon the solution into serving containers or small jars.

3. Put in the fridge for almost 2 hrs.

4. Top using fresh berries before serving if desired.

5. Present the lactose-free cheesecake bites.

Per serving: Calories: 300 kcal; Fat: 25g; Carbs: 15g; Protein: 5g; Fiber: 0g; Sodium: 200mg

147 - Frozen Grapes

Preparation time: 5 min.

Cooking time: 0 min.

Servings: 2

Ingredients:

- 2 cups seedless grapes (choose red or green)*
- Wooden skewers (elective)

Directions:

1. Wash the grapes and pat them dry.

2. Skewer the grapes onto wooden skewers or put them directly on a tray.

3. Freeze for almost 2 hrs.

4. Present the frozen grapes.

Per serving: Calories: 100 kcal; Fat: 0g; Carbs: 26g; Protein: 1g; Fiber: 2g; Sodium: 0mg

148 - Raspberry Almond Thumbprint Cookies

Preparation time: 15 min.

Cooking time: 10 min.

Servings: 2

Ingredients:

- 1 cup almond flour
- 2 tbsps maple syrup
- 1 tbsp coconut oil, dissolved
- 1/4 tsp almond extract
- 1/4 cup raspberry jam (low FODMAP)
- Sliced almonds for garnish

Directions:

1. Warm up the oven to 350 deg. F afterward, prepare your baking sheet by lining it with parchment paper.

2. In your container, mix almond flour, maple syrup, dissolved coconut oil, and almond extract until a dough forms.

3. Shape the dough into small balls and put them on to your prepared baking sheet.

4. Make an indentation in each cookie with your thumb.

5. Fill each indentation with a small amount of raspberry jam.

6. Garnish with carved almonds.

7. Bake for 10 min. or until the edges are golden.

8. Permit it to relax before serving.

9. Present the raspberry almond thumbprint cookies.

Per serving: Calories: 250 kcal; Fat: 18g; Carbs: 20g; Protein: 6g; Fiber: 3g; Sodium: 0mg

149 - Cantaloupe and Prosciutto Skewers

Preparation time: 10 min.

Cooking time: 0 min.

Servings: 2

Ingredients:

- 1/2 small cantaloupe, skinned and cut into cubes
- 4 slices prosciutto, cut into strips
- Wooden skewers

Directions:

1. Thread cantaloupe cubes and prosciutto strips alternately onto wooden skewers.

2. Organize the skewers on a serving plate.

3. Present the cantaloupe and prosciutto skewers.

Per serving: Calories: 150 kcal; Fat: 8g; Carbs: 15g; Protein: 8g; Fiber: 2g; Sodium: 800mg

150 - Chia Seed and Berry Parfait

Preparation time: 10 min.

Cooking time: 0 min.

Servings: 2

Ingredients:

- 1 cup lactose-free yogurt
- 2 tbsps chia seeds
- 1 cup Low FODMAP mixed berries (eg. blueberries)*
- 1 tbsp maple syrup (elective)
- Mint leaves for garnish

Directions:

1. In your container, mix lactose-free yogurt and chia seeds.

2. Put in the fridge for 1 hr to allow the chia seeds to expand.

3. In serving glasses, layer the chia seed solution with mixed berries.

4. Drizzle with maple syrup if desired.

5. Garnish with mint leaves.

6. Present the chia seed and berry parfait.

Per serving: Calories: 180 kcal; Fat: 8g; Carbs: 25g; Protein: 6g; Fiber: 8g; Sodium: 50mg

Sauces and Dressings Recipes

151 - Basil Pesto

Preparation time: 10 min.

Cooking time: 0 min.

Servings: 2

Ingredients:

- 2 cups fresh basil leaves
- 1/2 cup pine nuts
- 1/2 cup grated lactose-freeParmesan cheese
- 1/2 cup olive oil
- Salt and pepper as required
- Lemon juice as required

Directions:

1. In your blending container, blend basil leaves, pine nuts, and Parmesan cheese.

2. Pulse until finely chopped.

3. While your food processor is running, drizzle in the olive oil until the mixture forms a smooth paste.

4. Season with salt, pepper, and lemon juice as required.

5. Present the basil pesto over pasta, grilled chicken, or vegetables.

Per serving: Calories: 400 kcal; Fat: 38g; Carbs: 6g; Protein: 8g; Fiber: 2g; Sodium: 200mg

152 - Lemon Vinaigrette

Preparation time: 5 min.

Cooking time: 0 min.

Servings: 2

Ingredients:

- 1/4 cup olive oil
- 2 tbsps lemon juice
- 1 tsp Dijon mustard
- Salt and pepper as required

Directions:

1. In a mini container, whisk collectively Dijon mustard, olive oil, and lemon juice.

2. Season with salt and pepper as required.

3. Whisk until thoroughly blended.

4. Present the lemon vinaigrette over salads or grilled meats.

Per serving: Calories: 200 kcal; Fat: 20g; Carbs: 3g; Protein: 0g; Fiber: 0g; Sodium: 100mg

153 - Teriyaki Sauce (without garlic and onion)

Preparation time: 10 min.

Cooking time: 10 min.

Servings: 2

Ingredients:

- 1/2 cup soy sauce
- 1/4 cup brown sugar
- 2 tbsps rice vinegar
- 1 tsp fresh ginger, grated
- 1 tbsp chives, finely chopped (green part only)
- 1 tbsp sesame oil

Directions:

1. In a mini saucepot, blend soy sauce, brown sugar, rice vinegar, grated ginger, chopped chives, and sesame oil.

2. Heat over medium heat., stirring until the sugar dissolves.

3. Simmer for 8-10 min. or until the sauce thickens.

4. Permit it to relax before serving.

5. Present the teriyaki sauce over grilled chicken, tofu, or vegetables.

Per serving: Calories: 150 kcal; Fat: 7g; Carbs: 18g; Protein: 3g; Fiber: 0g; Sodium: 500mg

154 - Balsamic Glaze

Preparation time: 5 min.

Cooking time: 15 min.

Servings: 2

Ingredients:

- 1 cup balsamic vinegar*
- 2 tbsps maple syrup

Directions:

1. In a mini saucepot, blend balsamic vinegar and maple syrup.

2. Boil, then reduce the heat. to simmer.

3. Simmer for 15 min. or until the solution has reduced by half then has a syrupy consistency.

4. Permit it to relax before serving.

5. Present the balsamic glaze over salads, grilled meats, or vegetables.

Per serving: Calories: 150 kcal; Fat: 0g; Carbs: 36g; Protein: 0g; Fiber: 0g; Sodium: 20mg

155 - Chimichurri Sauce

Preparation time: 10 min.

Cooking time: 0 min.

Servings: 2

Ingredients:

- 1 cup fresh parsley, chopped
- 1/4 cup fresh cilantro, chopped
- 1 tsp dried oregano
- 1/2 tsp red pepper flakes
- 2 tbsps red wine vinegar
- 1/2 cup olive oil
- Salt and pepper as required

Directions:

1. In your container, blend dried oregano, chopped parsley, chopped cilantro, and red pepper flakes.

2. Include red wine vinegar and olive oil. Blend thoroughly.

3. Season with salt and pepper as required.

4. Allow the flavors to meld for almost 10 min. before serving.

5. Present the chimichurri sauce over grilled meats or vegetables.

Per serving: Calories: 350 kcal; Fat: 36g; Carbs: 4g; Protein: 1g; Fiber: 1g; Sodium: 10mg

156 - Maple Dijon Dressing

Preparation time: 5 min.

Cooking time: 0 min.

Servings: 2

Ingredients:

- 1/4 cup Dijon mustard
- 2 tbsps maple syrup
- 2 tbsps apple cider vinegar
- 1/4 cup olive oil
- Salt and pepper as required

Directions:

1. In a mini container, whisk collectively Dijon mustard, maple syrup, and apple cider vinegar.

2. Gradually whisk in olive oil until thoroughly blended.

3. Season with salt and pepper as required.

4. Present the maple Dijon dressing over salads or grilled meats.

Per serving: Calories: 250 kcal; Fat: 22g; Carbs: 14g; Protein: 1g; Fiber: 0g; Sodium: 280mg

157 - Tahini Yogurt Sauce

Preparation time: 5 min.

Cooking time: 0 min.

Servings: 2

Ingredients:

- 1/4 cup tahini
- 1/2 cup lactose-free yogurt
- 1 tbsp lemon juice
- 1 tbsp fresh parsley, chopped
- Salt and pepper as required

Directions:

1. In your container, whisk collectively tahini, lactose-free yogurt, lemon juice, and chopped parsley.

2. Season with salt and pepper as required.

3. Stir until thoroughly blended.

4. Serve the tahini yogurt sauce as a dip or drizzle it over grilled vegetables.

Per serving: Calories: 200 kcal; Fat: 16g; Carbs: 10g; Protein: 5g; Fiber: 1g; Sodium: 30mg

158 - Lactose-Free Ranch Dressing

Preparation time: 5 min.

Cooking time: 0 min.

Servings: 2

Ingredients:

- 1/2 cup lactose-free mayonnaise
- 1/2 cup lactose-free sour cream
- 1 tbsp fresh chives, chopped (green part only)
- 1 tbsp fresh parsley, chopped
- 1 tsp dried dill
- 1 tsp onion powder
- Salt and pepper as required

Directions:

1. In your container, whisk collectively lactose-free mayonnaise, lactose-free sour cream, chopped chives, chopped parsley, dried dill, and onion powder.

2. Season with salt and pepper as required.

3. Stir until thoroughly blended.

4. Present the lactose-free ranch dressing over salads or as a dip for vegetables.

Per serving: Calories: 300 kcal; Fat: 30g; Carbs: 4g; Protein: 1g; Fiber: 0g; Sodium: 250mg

159 - Olive Tapenade

Preparation time: 10 min.

Cooking time: 0 min.

Servings: 2

Ingredients:

- 1 cup Kalamata olives, eroded
- 2 tbsps capers
- 1 tbsp fresh parsley, chopped
- 1 tbsp lemon juice
- 2 tbsps extra virgin olive oil
- Black pepper as required

Directions:

1. In a blending container, blend Kalamata olives, capers, chopped parsley, and lemon juice.

2. Pulse until the solution is finely chopped.

3. While the processor is running, drizzle in the extra virgin olive oil.

4. Season with black pepper as required.

5. Allow the tapenade to sit for nearly 10 min. to let the flavors meld.

6. Present the olive tapenade as a spread on crackers or alongside grilled meats.

Per serving: Calories: 180 kcal; Fat: 18g; Carbs: 4g; Protein: 1g; Fiber: 2g; Sodium: 950mg

160 - Lemon Herb Marinade

Preparation time: 5 min.

Cooking time: 0 min.

Servings: 2

Ingredients:

- 1/4 cup fresh lemon juice
- 2 tbsps olive oil
- 1 tbsp fresh herbs (rosemary, thyme, or oregano), chopped
- 1 tsp Dijon mustard
- Salt and pepper as required

Directions:

1. In your container, whisk collectively fresh lemon juice, olive oil, chopped herbs, Dijon mustard, salt, and pepper.

2. Whisk until thoroughly blended.

3. Use the lemon herb marinade for marinating chicken, fish, or vegetables prior to grilling or roasting.

Per serving: Calories: 150 kcal; Fat: 14g; Carbs: 5g; Protein: 1g; Fiber: 0g; Sodium: 150mg

161 - Mango Salsa

Preparation time: 10 min.

Cooking time: 0 min.

Servings: 2

Ingredients:

- 1 ripe mango, cubed*
- 1/4 cup red bell pepper, cubed*
- 2 tbsps fresh cilantro, chopped
- 1 tbsp lime juice
- 1 tbsp green tops of green onions, chopped
- Salt and pepper as required

Directions:

1. In your container, blend cubed mango, cubed red bell pepper, chopped cilantro, lime juice, and chopped green onions.

2. Blend thoroughly.

3. Season with salt and pepper as required.

4. Allow the flavors to meld for almost 10 min. before serving.

5. Present your mango salsa as a topping for grilled chicken, fish, or tacos.

Per serving: Calories: 90 kcal; Fat: 0g; Carbs: 23g; Protein: 1g; Fiber: 3g; Sodium: 5mg

162 - Dill Sauce

Preparation time: 5 min.

Cooking time: 0 min.

Servings: 2

Ingredients:

- 1/2 cup lactose-free sour cream
- 2 tbsps fresh dill, chopped
- 1 tbsp lemon juice
- Salt and pepper as required

Directions:

1. In your container, blend collectively lactose-free sour cream, chopped fresh dill, and lemon juice.

2. Season with salt and pepper as required.

3. Stir until thoroughly blended.

4. Present the dill sauce as a condiment for grilled fish.

Per serving: Calories: 90 kcal; Fat: 8g; Carbs: 4g; Protein: 1g; Fiber: 0g; Sodium: 10mg

163 - Strawberry Balsamic Reduction

Preparation time: 5 min.

Cooking time: 15 min.

Servings: 2

Ingredients:

- 1 cup fresh strawberries, hulled and divided*
- 1/4 cup balsamic vinegar*
- 1 tbsp maple syrup (elective)

Directions:

1. In a mini saucepot, blend fresh strawberries, balsamic vinegar, and maple syrup (if using).

2. Simmer the solution over medium heat.

3. Reduce the heat to low and let it simmer for around 10-15 min. or until the strawberries are soft then the solution has thickened.

4. Allow the reduction to cool before serving.

5. Present the strawberry balsamic reduction over salads or grilled meats.

Per serving: Calories: 80 kcal; Fat: 0g; Carbs: 20g; Protein: 1g; Fiber: 3g; Sodium: 5mg

164 - Avocado Lime Dressing

Preparation time: 5 min.

Cooking time: 0 min.

Servings: 2

Ingredients:

- 1 ripe avocado, skinned and eroded
- 1/4 cup fresh cilantro, chopped
- 2 tbsps lime juice
- 2 tbsps olive oil
- Salt and pepper as required

Directions:

1. In a blender, blend ripe avocado, chopped cilantro, lime juice, and olive oil.

2. Blend until smooth.

3. Season with salt and pepper as required.

4. If too thick, you can thin it with a little water.

5. Present the avocado lime dressing over salads or grilled chicken.

Per serving: Calories: 200 kcal; Fat: 18g; Carbs: 10g; Protein: 2g; Fiber: 6g; Sodium: 10mg

165 - Tzatziki Sauce

Preparation time: 10 min.

Cooking time: 0 min.

Servings: 2

Ingredients:

- 1/2 cucumber, finely cubed
- 1 cup lactose-free Greek yogurt
- 1 tbsp fresh dill, chopped
- 1 tbsp lemon juice
- 1 tbsp olive oil
- Salt and pepper as required

Directions:

1. In your container, blend finely cubed cucumber, lactose-free Greek yogurt, chopped fresh dill, lemon juice, and olive oil.

2. Blend thoroughly.

3. Season with salt and pepper as required.

4. Allow the tzatziki sauce to chill in the fridge for 30 min. before serving.

5. Present the tzatziki sauce as a dip for vegetables or alongside grilled meats.

Per serving: Calories: 150 kcal; Fat: 10g; Carbs: 8g; Protein: 8g; Fiber: 1g; Sodium: 50mg

Juices Recipes

166 - Carrot and Orange Juice

Preparation time: 10 min.

Cooking time: 0 min.

Servings: 2

Ingredients:

- 4 medium carrots, skinned and chopped
- 2 oranges, skinned and segmented*
- 1 inch ginger, that is skinned and grated
- Ice cubes (elective)

Directions:

1. In a juicer, process the chopped carrots, segmented oranges, and grated ginger.

2. Pour the juice into glasses over ice cubes if desired.

3. Stir well before serving.

4. Present the carrot and orange juice chilled.

Per serving: Calories: 80 kcal; Fat: 0g; Carbs: 20g; Protein: 1g; Fiber: 4g; Sodium: 40mg

167 - Cucumber Mint Lemonade

Preparation time: 15 min.

Cooking time: 0 min.

Servings: 2

Ingredients:

- 1 cucumber, carved*
- 1/4 cup fresh mint leaves
- 2 lemons, juiced
- 2 tbsps maple syrup
- Ice cubes (elective)

Directions:

1. In a blender, blend cucumber slices, mint leaves, lemon juice, and maple syrup.

2. Blend until smooth.

3. Strain the solution to take out pulp if desired.

4. Pour the juice into glasses over ice cubes if desired.

5. Stir well before serving.

6. Present the cucumber mint lemonade chilled.

Per serving: Calories: 70 kcal; Fat: 0g; Carbs: 20g; Protein: 1g; Fiber: 2g; Sodium: 10mg

168 - Strawberry Kiwi Cooler

Preparation time: 10 min.

Cooking time: 0 min.

Servings: 2

Ingredients:

- 1 cup strawberries, hulled and divided*
- 2 kiwis, skinned and carved
- 1 tbsp lime juice
- 1 tbsp maple syrup
- Ice cubes (elective)

Directions:

1. In a blender, blend strawberries, kiwis, lime juice, and maple syrup.

2. Blend until smooth.

3. Strain the solution to take out seeds if desired.

4. Pour the juice into glasses over ice cubes if desired.

5. Stir well before serving.

6. Present the strawberry kiwi cooler chilled.

Per serving: Calories: 80 kcal; Fat: 0g; Carbs: 20g; Protein: 1g; Fiber: 3g; Sodium: 5mg

169 - Pineapple Ginger Turmeric Juice

Preparation time: 15 min.

Cooking time: 0 min.

Servings: 2

Ingredients:

- 1 cup fresh pineapple chunks*
- 1 inch ginger, that is skinned and grated
- 1/2 tsp ground turmeric
- 1 tbsp honey*
- Ice cubes (elective)

Directions:

1. In a juicer, process the pineapple chunks, grated ginger, ground turmeric, and honey.

2. Pour the juice into glasses over ice cubes if desired.

3. Stir well before serving.

4. Present the pineapple ginger turmeric juice chilled.

Per serving: Calories: 90 kcal; Fat: 0g; Carbs: 25g; Protein: 1g; Fiber: 2g; Sodium: 0mg

170 - Green Apple and Spinach Juice

Preparation time: 10 min.

Cooking time: 0 min.

Servings: 2

Ingredients:

- 2 green apples, cored and carved*
- 2 cups fresh spinach leaves
- 1/2 cucumber, carved*
- 1 lemon, juiced
- Ice cubes (elective)

Directions:

1. In a juicer, process the green apples, spinach leaves, cucumber slices, and lemon juice.

2. Pour the juice into glasses over ice cubes if desired.

3. Stir well before serving.

4. Present the green apple and spinach juice chilled.

Per serving: Calories: 80 kcal; Fat: 0g; Carbs: 20g; Protein: 2g; Fiber: 5g; Sodium: 20mg

171 - Watermelon Cucumber Refresher

Preparation time: 10 min.

Cooking time: 0 min.

Servings: 2

Ingredients:

- 2 cups watermelon, cubed
- 1/2 cucumber, carved*
- 1 tbsp lime juice
- 1 tbsp fresh mint leaves
- Ice cubes (elective)

Directions:

1. In a blender, blend cubed watermelon, cucumber slices, lime juice, and fresh mint leaves.

2. Blend until smooth.

3. Strain the solution to take out pulp if desired.

4. Pour the juice into glasses over ice cubes if desired.

5. Stir well before serving.

6. Present the watermelon cucumber refresher chilled.

Per serving: Calories: 50 kcal; Fat: 0g; Carbs: 15g; Protein: 1g; Fiber: 1g; Sodium: 5mg

172 - Blueberry Lemonade

Preparation time: 10 min.

Cooking time: 0 min.

Servings: 2

Ingredients:

- 1 cup blueberries
- 2 lemons, juiced
- 2 tbsps maple syrup
- 2 cups cold water
- Ice cubes (elective)

Directions:

1. In a blender, blend blueberries, lemon juice, maple syrup, and cold water.

2. Blend until smooth.

3. Strain the solution to take out pulp if desired.

4. Pour the blueberry lemonade into glasses over ice cubes if desired.

5. Stir well before serving.

6. Present the blueberry lemonade chilled.

Per serving: Calories: 80 kcal; Fat: 0g; Carbs: 20g; Protein: 1g; Fiber: 3g; Sodium: 5mg

173 - Beet and Berry Blast

Preparation time: 15 min.

Cooking time: 0 min.

Servings: 2

Ingredients:

- 1 small beet, skinned and cubed
- 1 cup Low FODMAP mixed berries (eg. blueberries)*
- 1 tbsp lemon juice
- 1 tbsp honey*
- 2 cups cold water
- Ice cubes (elective)

Directions:

1. In a blender, blend cubed beet, mixed berries, lemon juice, honey, and cold water.

2. Blend until smooth.

3. Strain the solution to take out pulp if desired.

4. Pour the beet and berry blast into glasses over ice cubes if desired.

5. Stir well before serving.

6. Present the beet and berry blast chilled.

Per serving: Calories: 90 kcal; Fat: 0g; Carbs: 25g; Protein: 1g; Fiber: 5g; Sodium: 30mg

174 - Mango Pineapple Mint Smoothie

Preparation time: 10 min.

Cooking time: 0 min.

Servings: 2

Ingredients:

- 1 cup fresh or frozen mango chunks*
- 1 cup fresh or frozen pineapple chunks*
- 1 tbsp lime juice
- 1 tbsp fresh mint leaves
- 1 cup coconut water
- Ice cubes (elective)

Directions:

1. In a blender, blend mango chunks, pineapple chunks, lime juice, fresh mint leaves, and coconut water.

2. Blend until smooth.

3. Pour the smoothie into glasses over ice cubes if desired.

4. Stir well before serving.

5. Present the mango pineapple mint smoothie chilled.

Per serving: Calories: 120 kcal; Fat: 1g; Carbs: 30g; Protein: 2g; Fiber: 4g; Sodium: 70mg

175 - Kiwi and Kale Green Juice

Preparation time: 10 min.

Cooking time: 0 min.

Servings: 2

Ingredients:

- 2 kiwis, skinned and carved
- 1 cup kale leaves, stems taken out
- 1 cucumber, carved*
- 1 lemon, juiced
- 1 tbsp honey*
- 2 cups cold water
- Ice cubes (elective)

Directions:

1. In a juicer, process kiwi slices, kale leaves, cucumber slices, lemon juice, honey, and cold water.

2. Pour the green juice into glasses over ice cubes if desired.

3. Stir well before serving.

4. Present the kiwi and kale green juice chilled.

Per serving: Calories: 70 kcal; Fat: 0g; Carbs: 20g; Protein: 2g; Fiber: 4g; Sodium: 20mg

176 - Citrus Berry Punch

Preparation time: 10 min.

Cooking time: 0 min.

Servings: 2

Ingredients:

• 1 cup Low FODMAP mixed berries (eg. blueberries)*
• 1 orange, skinned and segmented*
• 1/2 grapefruit, skinned and segmented*
• 1 tbsp lime juice
• 2 tbsps maple syrup
• 2 cups cold water
• Ice cubes (elective)

Directions:

1. In a blender, blend mixed berries, orange segments, grapefruit segments, lime juice, maple syrup, and cold water.

2. Blend until smooth.

3. Strain the solution to take out pulp if desired.

4. Pour the citrus berry punch into glasses over ice cubes if desired.

5. Stir well before serving.

6. Present the citrus berry punch chilled.

Per serving: Calories: 80 kcal; Fat: 0g; Carbs: 20g; Protein: 1g; Fiber: 4g; Sodium: 10mg

177 - Papaya Lime Splash

Preparation time: 10 min.

Cooking time: 0 min.

Servings: 2

Ingredients:

• 1 cup ripe papaya, cubed
• 1 lime, juiced
• 1 tbsp honey*
• 2 cups cold water
• Ice cubes (elective)

Directions:

1. In a blender, blend cubed papaya, lime juice, honey, and cold water.

2. Blend until smooth.

3. Strain the solution to take out pulp if desired.

4. Pour the papaya lime splash into glasses over ice cubes if desired.

5. Stir well before serving.

6. Present the papaya lime splash chilled.

Per serving: Calories: 80 kcal; Fat: 0g; Carbs: 20g; Protein: 1g; Fiber: 2g; Sodium: 5mg

178 - Ginger Pear Juice

Preparation time: 15 min.

Cooking time: 0 min.

Servings: 2

Ingredients:

- 2 Nashi pears, skinned and carved*
- 1-inch ginger, that is skinned and grated
- 1 tbsp lemon juice
- 1 tbsp honey
- 2 cups cold water
- Ice cubes (elective)

Directions:

1. In a juicer, process carved pears, grated ginger, lemon juice, honey, and cold water.

2. Pour the ginger pear juice into glasses over ice cubes if desired.

3. Stir well before serving.

4. Present the ginger pear juice chilled.

Per serving: Calories: 90 kcal; Fat: 0g; Carbs: 25g; Protein: 1g; Fiber: 5g; Sodium: 0mg

179 - Cranberry Lime Spritzer

Preparation time: 10 min.

Cooking time: 0 min.

Servings: 2

Ingredients:

- 1/2 cup cranberry juice (unsweetened)
- 1 lime, juiced
- 2 tbsps maple syrup
- 2 cups sparkling water
- Ice cubes (elective)

Directions:

1. In a pitcher, blend cranberry juice, lime juice, maple syrup, and sparkling water.

2. Stir well until the components are mixed.

3. Pour the cranberry lime spritzer into glasses over ice cubes if desired.

4. Stir well before serving.

5. Present the cranberry lime spritzer chilled.

Per serving: Calories: 50 kcal; Fat: 0g; Carbs: 15g; Protein: 0g; Fiber: 0g; Sodium: 0mg

180 - Orange Basil Mocktail

Preparation time: 10 min.

Cooking time: 0 min.

Servings: 2

Ingredients:

- 1 cup fresh orange juice
- 1 tbsp fresh basil leaves, chopped
- 2 tbsps maple syrup
- 2 cups cold water
- Ice cubes (elective)

Directions:

1. In a blender, blend fresh orange juice, chopped basil leaves, maple syrup, and cold water.

2. Blend until smooth.

3. Strain the solution to take out pulp if desired.

4. Pour the orange basil mocktail into glasses over ice cubes if desired.

5. Stir well before serving.

6. Present the orange basil mocktail chilled.

Per serving: Calories: 70 kcal; Fat: 0g; Carbs: 20g; Protein: 1g; Fiber: 1g; Sodium: 5mg

CHAPTER 4: Comprehensive Support Resources

An 8-Week Meal Plan Ready for You

This 8-week meal plan is structured to guide you through the different phases of the Low FODMAP Diet. Each week includes a recipes for breakfast, lunch, dinner and dessert ideas. It's important to note that this meal plan is a general guide, and individual tolerance to specific FODMAPs may vary.

Week 1:

Day	Breakfast	Lunch	Dinner	Dessert
1	Peanut Butter Banana Toast (13)	Turkey and Cranberry Quinoa Stuffed Peppers (51)	Lemon Herb Baked Chicken (61)	Dark Chocolate-Dipped Strawberries (122)
2	Blueberry Oat Pancakes (4)	Salmon and Avocado Sushi Rolls (38)	Beef and Broccoli Stir-Fry (62)	Mango and Lime Sorbet (135)
3	Chia Seed Pudding with Kiwi (5)	Quinoa and Grilled Chicken Bowl (32)	Grilled Swordfish with Citrus Salsa (63)	Rice Cake with Peanut Butter and Banana (124)
4	Avocado and Bacon Breakfast Sandwich (16)	Shrimp and Mango Lettuce Wraps (52)	Ratatouille with Herbed Quinoa (64)	Lactose-Free Vanilla Pudding with Berries (131)
5	Maple Pecan Granola with Lactose-Free Yogurt (25)	Egg Salad Lettuce Wraps (47)	Lactose-Free Spinach and Feta Stuffed Portobello Mushrooms (65)	Kiwi and Pineapple Fruit Salad (129)
6	Greek Yogurt Parfait with Strawberries (9)	Quinoa Salad with Roasted Vegetables (48)	Pork and Pineapple Skewers (66)	Chocolate Avocado Mousse (126)
7	Kiwi and Strawberry Breakfast Salad (21)	Lemon Herb Chicken Skewers (40)	Shrimp Scampi with Zucchini Noodles (67)	Maple Cinnamon Roasted Nuts (127)

Week 2:

Day	Breakfast	Lunch	Dinner	Dessert
1	Orange Ginger Turmeric Smoothie (28)	Lactose-Free Margherita Pizza (44)	Zoodle Carbonara with Bacon and Peas (72)	Strawberry and Kiwi Popsicles (138)
2	Rice Cake with Smoked Turkey and Tomato (24)	Teriyaki Tofu and Broccoli Stir-Fry (46)	Lemon Dill Salmon with Roasted Potatoes (71)	Lactose-Free Cheesecake Bites (146)
3	Coconut Flour Banana Muffins (23)	Quinoa Salad with Roasted Vegetables (48)	Grilled Chicken Caesar Salad (78)	Chocolate Banana Smoothie (145)
4	Frittata with Sun-Dried Tomatoes and Basil (20)	Lemon Dill Salmon Patties (59)	Mediterranean Baked Cod (68)	Roasted Chickpeas with Paprika (140)
5	Scrambled Eggs with Spinach and Tomatoes (1)	Lactose-Free Caprese Salad (36)	Grilled Vegetable and Polenta Stack (50)	Popcorn with Olive Oil and Herbs (132)
6	Banana Almond Butter Smoothie (6)	Tuna Salad with Cucumber and Olives (33)	Zucchini and Tomato Gratin (89)	Greek Yogurt with Honey and Walnuts (137)
7	Polenta and Vegetable Breakfast Skillet (10)	Shrimp and Avocado Salad (42)	Seared Scallops with Garlic Butter (85)	Lactose-Free Ice Cream with Chocolate Sauce (136)

Week 3:

Day	Breakfast	Lunch	Dinner	Dessert
1	Zucchini and Feta Omelet (7)	Quinoa Salad with Roasted Vegetables (48)	Stuffed Acorn Squash with Quinoa and Cranberries (81)	Grapes and Cheese Kabobs (128)
2	Pineapple Mango Smoothie Bowl (17)	Egg Salad Lettuce Wraps (47)	Pesto Zoodle Bowl with Cherry Tomatoes (72)	Nut and Seed Bars (139)
3	Cinnamon Raisin Overnight Oats (8)	Teriyaki Chicken and Vegetable Skillet (73)	Lactose-Free Margherita Zucchini Boats (82)	Lemon Sorbet with Mint (142)
4	Rice Cake with Avocado and Cherry Tomatoes (143)	Lemony Chicken and Rice Bowl (49)	Baked Cod with Lemon and Dill (84)	Almond and Pumpkin Seed Trail Mix (121)
5	Gluten-Free Buckwheat Waffles (15)	Grilled Pork Chops with Pineapple Salsa (43)	Seared Tofu with Peanut Sauce (57)	Raspberry Almond Thumbprint Cookies (148)
6	Quiche with Spinach and Lactose-Free Cheese (18)	Turkey and Zucchini Burgers (55)	Grilled Lamb Chops with Mint Chimichurri (90)	Lactose-Free Ice Cream with Chocolate Sauce (136)
7	Hash Browns with Bell Peppers and Eggs (29)	Quinoa and Grilled Chicken Bowl (32)	Zoodle Carbonara with Bacon and Peas (72)	Maple Cinnamon Roasted Nuts (127)

Week 4:

Day	Breakfast	Lunch	Dinner	Dessert
1	Kiwi and Strawberry Breakfast Salad (21)	Mediterranean Stuffed Bell Peppers (37)	Grilled Swordfish with Citrus Salsa (63)	Chocolate Avocado Mousse (126)
2	Orange Ginger Turmeric Smoothie (28)	Lactose-Free Margherita Pizza (44)	Beef and Broccoli Stir-Fry (62)	Kiwi and Pineapple Fruit Salad (129)
3	Quinoa Breakfast Bowl with Berries (2)	Salmon and Avocado Sushi Rolls (38)	Lactose-Free Spinach and Feta Stuffed Portobello Mushrooms (65)	Dark Chocolate-Dipped Strawberries (122)
4	Rice Cake with Smoked Turkey and Tomato (24)	Shrimp and Mango Lettuce Wraps (52)	Ratatouille with Herbed Quinoa (64)	Lactose-Free Vanilla Pudding with Berries (131)
5	Banana Almond Butter Smoothie (6)	Teriyaki Tofu and Broccoli Stir-Fry (46)	Lemon Dill Salmon with Roasted Potatoes (71)	Strawberry and Kiwi Popsicles (138)
6	Chia Seed Pudding with Kiwi (5)	Tuna Salad with Cucumber and Olives (33)	Grilled Vegetable and Polenta Stack (50)	Maple Cinnamon Roasted Nuts (127)
7	Polenta and Vegetable Breakfast Skillet (10)	Shrimp and Avocado Salad (42)	Seared Scallops with Garlic Butter (85)	Lactose-Free Ice Cream with Chocolate Sauce (136)

Week 5:

Day	Breakfast	Lunch	Dinner	Dessert
1	Scrambled Eggs with Spinach and Tomatoes (1)	Turkey and Cranberry Lettuce Wraps (31)	Lemon Herb Baked Chicken (61)	Almond and Pumpkin Seed Trail Mix (121)
2	Quinoa Breakfast Bowl with Berries (2)	Grilled Shrimp and Vegetable Skewers (34)	Zoodle Carbonara With Bacon and Peas (72)	Dark Chocolate-Dipped Strawberries (122)
3	Peanut Butter Banana Toast (13)	Lactose-Free Caprese Salad (36)	Pork and Pineapple Skewers (66)	Lactose-Free Yogurt with Berries (123)
4	Kiwi And Strawberry Breakfast Salad (21)	Egg Salad Lettuce Wraps (47)	Shrimp Scampi with Zucchini Noodles (67)	Rice Cake with Peanut Butter and Banana (124)
5	Maple Pecan Granola with Lactose-Free Yogurt (25)	Quinoa Salad with Roasted Vegetables (48)	Mediterranean Baked Cod (68)	Orange Slices with Tajin (125)
6	Greek Yogurt Parfait with Strawberries (9)	Grilled Vegetable and Polenta Stack (50)	Chicken and Vegetable Kebabs (69)	Chocolate Avocado Mousse (126)
7	Rice Cake with Smoked Turkey and Tomato (24)	Teriyaki Tofu and Broccoli Stir-Fry (46)	Zucchini and Tomato Gratin (89)	Maple Cinnamon Roasted Nuts (127)

Week 6:

Day	Breakfast	Lunch	Dinner	Dessert
1	Sweet Potato Hash with Poached Eggs	Lemon Herb Chicken Skewers (40)	Baked Turkey Meatballs with Zucchini Noodles (76)	Grapes and Cheese Kabobs (128)
2	Quiche with Spinach and Lactose-Free Cheese (14)	Zucchini Noodles with Pesto and Cherry Tomatoes (41)	Pan-Seared Steak with Chimichurri Sauce (77)	Kiwi and Pineapple Fruit Salad (129)
3	Frittata with Sun-Dried Tomatoes and Basil (20)	Grilled Pork Chops with Pineapple Salsa (43)	Grilled Chicken Caesar Salad (78)	Peanut Butter Energy Bites (130)
4	Gluten-Free Buckwheat Waffles (15)	Beef and Vegetable Lettuce Cups (45)	Spaghetti Squash with Tomato Basil Sauce (79)	Lactose-Free Vanilla Pudding with Berries (131)
5	Pineapple Mango Smoothie Bowl (17)	Turkey and Cranberry Quinoa Stuffed Peppers (51)	Pesto Zucchini Noodles with Grilled Chicken (80)	Popcorn with Olive Oil and Herbs (132)
6	Avocado and Bacon Breakfast Sandwich (16)	Shrimp and Mango Lettuce Wraps (52)	Stuffed Acorn Squash with Quinoa and Cranberries (81)	Rice Crackers with Smoked Salmon (133)
7	Cinnamon Raisin Overnight Oats (8)	Lactose-Free Greek Salad (53)	Lactose-Free Margherita Zucchini Boats (82)	Dark Chocolate Almond Clusters (134)

Week 7:

Day	Breakfast	Lunch	Dinner	Dessert
1	Coconut Flour Banana Muffins (23)	Pesto Zoodle Bowl with Cherry Tomatoes (54)	Lemon Dill Salmon with Roasted Potatoes (71)	Mango and Lime Sorbet (135)
2	Zucchini and Feta Omelet (7)	Turkey and Zucchini Burgers (55)	Zoodle Carbonara With Bacon and Peas (72)	Lactose-Free Ice Cream with Chocolate Sauce (136)
3	Orange Ginger Turmeric Smoothie (28)	Roasted Red Pepper & Goat Cheese Stuffed Chicken (56)	Teriyaki Chicken and Vegetable Skillet (73)	Greek Yogurt with Honey and Walnuts (137)
4	Hash Browns with Bell Peppers and Eggs (29)	Seared Tofu with Peanut Sauce (57)	Lactose-Free Margherita Risotto (74)	Strawberry and Kiwi Popsicles (138)
5	Kiwi And Strawberry Breakfast Salad (21)	Chicken and Quinoa Spring Rolls (58)	Maple Glazed Salmon with Roasted Brussels Sprouts (75)	Nut and Seed Bars (139)
6	Rice Cake with Smoked Turkey and Tomato (24)	Lemon Dill Salmon Patties (59)	Baked Cod with Lemon and Dill (84)	Roasted Chickpeas with Paprika (140)
7	Blueberry Oat Pancakes (4)	Vegetable and Rice Paper Rolls (60)	Seared Scallops with Garlic Butter (85)	Pineapple Coconut Chia Pudding (141)

Week 8:

Day	Breakfast	Lunch	Dinner	Dessert
1	Polenta and Vegetable Breakfast Skillet (10)	Lemon Dill Salmon Patties (59)	Grilled Lamb Chops with Mint Chimichurri (90)	Lemon Sorbet with Mint (142)
2	Omelet with Bell Peppers and Goat Cheese (11)	Salmon and Avocado Sushi Rolls (38)	Grilled Swordfish with Citrus Salsa (63)	Rice Cake with Avocado and Cherry Tomatoes (143)
3	Low Fodmap Breakfast Burrito (22)	Spinach and Feta Stuffed Chicken Breast (39)	Ratatouille with Herbed Quinoa (64)	Blueberry Almond Granola Bars (144)
4	Spinach and Tomato Breakfast Quesadilla (12)	Lactose-Free Margherita Pizza (44)	Chicken and Vegetable Kebabs (69)	Chocolate Banana Smoothie (145)
5	Peanut Butter Banana Toast (13)	Tuna Salad with Cucumber and Olives (33)	Grilled Chicken Caesar Salad (78)	Lactose-Free Cheesecake Bites (146)
6	Greek Yogurt Parfait with Strawberries (9)	Zucchini Noodles with Pesto and Cherry Tomatoes (41)	Eggplant Parmesan with Gluten-Free Breadcrumbs (70)	Frozen Grapes (147)
7	Papaya and Lime Breakfast Boat (30)	Beef and Vegetable Lettuce Cups (45)	Stuffed Acorn Squash with Quinoa and Cranberries (81)	Raspberry Almond Thumbprint Cookies (148)

20 Most Frequently Asked Questions and Concerns

Navigating the Low FODMAP journey comes with various questions and concerns. Here are answers to 20 frequently asked questions, addressing common uncertainties and providing guidance for individuals managing Irritable Bowel Syndrome (IBS) through this dietary approach:

1. What if I accidentally consume high-FODMAP foods?

Accidental consumption may occur, but it's essential not to panic. Monitor symptoms, and if a reaction occurs, focus on returning to a low FODMAP diet. Learn from the experience to prevent future incidents.

2. How long will it take to see improvements in my symptoms?

Individual responses vary. Some may experience relief within a couple of weeks, while others may need more time. Patience is key, and consistent adherence to the Low FODMAP Diet is crucial for optimal results.

3. Can I ever reintroduce my favorite high-FODMAP foods back into my diet?

Yes, the reintroduction phase allows systematic reintroduction of specific FODMAP groups to identify personal triggers. With a dietitian's guidance, you can reintroduce and assess tolerance.

4. How do I handle social situations like dining out or attending parties?

Plan ahead by researching menus, sharing dietary needs with hosts or restaurants, and bringing Low FODMAP snacks to social events. Being proactive ensures enjoyable social experiences.

5. Is the Low FODMAP Diet a lifelong commitment?

No, the diet is not meant to be lifelong. After identifying trigger FODMAPs, you can reintroduce well-tolerated foods, creating a more varied and sustainable long-term eating plan.

6. Can I follow a vegetarian or vegan Low FODMAP Diet?

Yes, a vegetarian or vegan Low FODMAP Diet is possible. Consult with a dietitian to ensure nutritional adequacy, as some high-protein plant sources are also high in FODMAPs.

7. Are there Low FODMAP alternatives for gluten-free diets?

Yes, many gluten-free alternatives are Low FODMAP. Examples include rice, quinoa, and gluten-free oats. Check labels for hidden FODMAPs in gluten-free products.

8. Can I use artificial sweeteners on the Low FODMAP Diet?

Some artificial sweeteners are low in FODMAPs and can be used in moderation. Examples include stevia and aspartame. However, others like sorbitol and mannitol are high FODMAP and should be avoided.

9. How do I manage fiber intake on the Low FODMAP Diet?

Focus on low FODMAP, high-fiber foods such as carrots, zucchini, and gluten-free oats. Gradually increase fiber intake and stay hydrated to support digestive health.

10. Can I drink alcohol on the Low FODMAP Diet?

Certain alcoholic beverages are low in FODMAPs, such as dry wine and some spirits. However, beer and certain sweet wines may be high in FODMAPs and should be consumed with caution. Therefore, if you would like a beer, ensure it is a Low Fodmap one before.

11. What are some low FODMAP options for snacks?

Low FODMAP snacks include hard cheeses, rice cakes, nuts in moderation (e.g., almonds, walnuts), and fresh fruits like strawberries and blueberries.

12. How do I handle travel while on the Low FODMAP Diet?

Plan snacks and meals in advance, research dining options at your destination, and bring portable Low FODMAP snacks. Staying prepared ensures dietary adherence during travel.

13. Can stress impact IBS symptoms on the Low FODMAP Diet?

Yes, stress can exacerbate IBS symptoms. Incorporate stress-management techniques such as mindfulness and relaxation exercises into your routine.

14. Can I use garlic and onion substitutes in cooking?

Yes, garlic-infused oil is a suitable substitute for garlic, and infused oils with low FODMAP herbs can replace onion in recipes.

15. Can I consume lactose-free dairy on the Low FODMAP Diet?

Yes, lactose-free dairy products are generally well-tolerated. However, some individuals may still be sensitive, so monitor individual responses.

16. Are there specific probiotics recommended for IBS on the Low FODMAP Diet?

Some probiotics may offer symptom relief, but in the elimination phase they can make it difficult to pinpoint the triggers. Consult with a healthcare professional to find the best option for you.

17. Can I use high FODMAP ingredients in small amounts?

Portion control is essential. Small amounts of some high FODMAP components may be tolerated. Experiment cautiously and monitor responses.

18. How do I handle cravings for high FODMAP foods?

Find Low FODMAP alternatives for your favorite flavors. Experiment with recipes to recreate familiar tastes without triggering symptoms.

19. What if I have other dietary restrictions in addition to Low FODMAP?

A registered dietitian can help create a customized eating plan considering multiple dietary restrictions to ensure optimal nutritional intake.

20. Can children follow the Low FODMAP Diet?

The Low FODMAP Diet may not be suitable for children without proper supervision. Consult with a pediatric dietitian to explore appropriate dietary strategies for children with digestive issues.

Apps, Tools for Tracking, Further Reading, Support Groups

Navigating the Low FODMAP journey becomes more manageable with the aid of modern technology, comprehensive resources, and supportive communities. Here are valuable apps, tools, reading materials, and support groups to enhance your experience:

1. **Monash University FODMAP App:** Developed by Monash University, this app is a comprehensive guide for identifying FODMAP content in foods. It provides up-to-date information on low and high FODMAP foods, serving sizes, and a food diary for tracking.

2. **FODMAP Friendly App:** This app offers a user-friendly interface to identify FODMAP levels in various foods. It includes a barcode scanner for easy product checking and a meal planner.

3. **MySymptoms App:** Ideal for tracking symptoms, food intake, and stress levels. This app helps users correlate their diet and lifestyle with symptom occurrences.

4. **Low FODMAP Diet by Kate Scarlata and Dedé Wilson:** Kate Scarlata, a registered dietitian, and Dedé Wilson offer a comprehensive book on the Low FODMAP Diet. It provides practical advice, recipes, and insights into managing IBS symptoms.

5. **"The Complete Low-FODMAP Diet" by Sue Shepherd and Peter Gibson:** Authored by pioneers in FODMAP research, this book offers a detailed guide to the diet, including recipes, meal plans, and strategies for long-term success.

6. **Monash University FODMAP Blog:** The Monash University FODMAP Blog is a valuable resource for staying updated on the latest research, recipes, and tips related to the Low FODMAP Diet.

7. **Low FODMAP Recipes Websites:** Explore websites like FODMAP Everyday, A Little Bit Yummy, and Kate Scarlata's blog for a variety of Low FODMAP recipes, meal ideas, and cooking tips.

8. **Casa de Sante:** Casa de Sante offers Low FODMAP certified products, including seasonings and spice blends. Their website provides recipes and resources for a flavorful Low FODMAP experience.

9. **Join the Low FODMAP Diet Support Group on Facebook:** This Facebook group connects individuals on the Low FODMAP journey. Members share experiences, recipe ideas, and offer support and encouragement.

10. **Irritable Bowel Syndrome (IBS) Self Help and Support Group:** A supportive community on Reddit, this group is not only focused on the Low FODMAP Diet but also covers various aspects of managing IBS, including emotional well-being.

11. **FODMAP Life Community:** Created by a FODMAP-trained registered dietitian, this community offers resources, recipes, and a platform for individuals to share their Low FODMAP experiences.

12. **The Gut Foundation:** The Gut Foundation provides information on gut health, including resources on the Low FODMAP Diet. It's a valuable source for understanding the connection between diet and digestive health.

13. **FODMAP Everyday Podcast:** This podcast explores various aspects of the Low FODMAP Diet, featuring experts, success stories, and practical advice for integrating the diet into daily life.

14. **Pinterest Low FODMAP Boards:** Search for Low FODMAP boards on Pinterest for a wealth of recipe ideas, meal plans, and lifestyle tips shared by the community.

15. **FODMAP Travel and Lifestyle Bloggers:** Follow bloggers like Erin from Erin Lives Whole or Alana Scott, The FODMAP Challenge, for personal insights, travel tips, and lifestyle advice while on the Low FODMAP Diet.

Integrating these apps, tools, reading materials, and support groups into your Low FODMAP journey can enhance your understanding, provide practical solutions, and connect you with a supportive community facing similar challenges. Remember to consult with healthcare professionals and registered dietitians for personalized guidance on your journey.

Global Kitchen Measurement Units and Their Equivalents

Measurement Unit	Equivalent in Grams	Commonly Used In
Gram (g)	1 g	Globally
Ounce (oz)	28.35 g	US, UK
Pound (lb)	453.59 g	US, UK
Tablespoon (tbsp)	Approx. 15 g	US, Canada, Australia
Teaspoon (tsp)	Approx. 5 g	US, Canada, Australia
Cup (cup)	Approx. 240 g	US, Canada
Pint (pt)	473.18 g	US, UK
Quart (qt)	946.35 g	US, UK
Liter (l)	1000 g	Globally

CHAPTER 5: Conclusion and Moving Forward

As you reach the culmination of your Low FODMAP journey, it's time to reflect on the strides you've made, the lessons learned, and the empowerment gained in the pursuit of better digestive health. The journey may have presented challenges, but it has also equipped you with valuable tools to navigate the intricate landscape of Irritable Bowel Syndrome (IBS). This concluding chapter serves as a guide to embracing your new lifestyle and forging a path towards sustained digestive well-being.

Embracing Your New Lifestyle

As you step into this new chapter of embracing your transformed lifestyle, it's time to reflect on the lessons learned, celebrate your successes, and move forward with confidence towards sustained digestive well-being. Here's a guide to help you navigate the path of embracing your new lifestyle:

• **Celebrating Successes:** Take a moment to acknowledge and celebrate the successes, both big and small, that you've achieved during your Low FODMAP journey. Whether it's identifying trigger foods, mastering meal planning, or confidently navigating social situations, each triumph contributes to your overall success.
• **Mindful Eating Practices:** Embrace mindful eating as a key aspect of your new lifestyle. Be present during meals, savor the flavors of Low FODMAP foods, and pay attention to your body's responses. Mindful eating fosters a positive relationship with food and enhances overall well-being.
• **Flexibility and Adaptability:** Understand that the Low FODMAP Diet is not static. It evolves with your growing awareness of your body's responses. Be open to adjustments and embrace the flexibility that comes with personalizing your dietary approach.

The Path to Better Digestive Health

Your journey toward better digestive health is a testament to your commitment to well-being and resilience in the face of challenges. As you move forward, consider the following steps to continue forging a path toward sustained digestive health:

• **Continued Guidance:** Maintain a connection with healthcare professionals, especially your registered dietitian. Regular check-ins and ongoing guidance ensure that you stay on the path to better digestive health with confidence and support.
• **Long-Term Sustainability:** Recognize that the journey towards better digestive health is an ongoing process. The skills and knowledge acquired during the Low FODMAP journey present as a foundation for a sustainable, long-term approach to managing IBS symptoms.
• **Integration of High-FODMAP Foods:** As you progress, you may explore reintroducing some of your favorite high-FODMAP foods. The reintroduction phase is a dynamic process, allowing you to discern your individual tolerances and expand the variety in your diet.

In conclusion, remember that you are equipped not only with the knowledge of the Low FODMAP Diet but also with a deeper understanding of your body and its unique responses. Embrace the lessons learned, celebrate your victories, and move forward with the confidence that comes from taking charge of your digestive health. Your journey is a testament to resilience, adaptability, and the transformative power of self-care. As you step into this new chapter, may it be marked by continued growth, sustained well-being, and a flourishing sense of empowerment.

CHAPTER 6: Term Glossary

Celiac Disease: An autoimmune disorder triggered by the ingestion of gluten, leading to damage in the small intestine.

Digestive Disorders: Conditions affecting the digestive system, including gastroesophageal reflux disease (GERD), inflammatory bowel disease (IBD), irritable bowel syndrome (IBS), etc.

Digestive System: Also referred to as the gastrointestinal (GI) tract, it is the intricate system tasked with the breakdown of food into nutrients, absorption of these nutrients, and the elimination of waste. Key organs within this system include the stomach, small intestine, and big intestine.

Efficient Digestion: The process by which the digestive system breaks down food into smaller, absorbable components through mechanical and chemical processes.

Elimination Phase: The initial phase of the Low FODMAP Diet where high-FODMAP foods are restricted to identify trigger foods.

Fermentable Oligosaccharides, Disaccharides, Monosaccharides, and Polyols (FODMAPs): Types of poorly immersed carbohydrates that can trigger symptoms in individuals with IBS. Found in certain foods, they ferment in the colon, leading to gas and other symptoms.

Functional Disorder: A disorder where the organs appear normal but do not function properly. IBS is an example of a functional disorder.

Gut Microbiota Balance: The balance of microorganisms in the digestive tract, crucial for digestion, nutrient absorption, and immune system function.

Inflammatory Bowel Disease (IBD): Chronic inflammatory conditions of the digestive tract, including Crohn's disease and ulcerative colitis.

Low FODMAP Diet: A dietary approach to manage IBS symptoms by reducing the intake of specific FODMAPs. It involves three phases: elimination, reintroduction, and personalization.

Metabolic Health: The interconnectedness of digestive and metabolic functions, emphasizing the importance of maintaining a healthy weight for overall well-being.

Monash University: It is the pioneering institution behind the Low FODMAP diet, researching and providing extensive resources to manage gastrointestinal disorders like IBS. Their work includes identifying FODMAP content in foods and developing diet strategies.

Nutrient Absorption: The small intestine's role in absorbing nutrients, including carbohydrates, proteins, fats, vitamins, and minerals, into the bloodstream for use by the body.

Personalization Phase: Follows reintroduction, involving a modified diet that limits only specific trigger FODMAPs, creating a personalized and sustainable approach.

Registered Dietitian: A professional with expertise in nutritional science, providing guidance on dietary strategies, including the Low FODMAP Diet.

Regular Bowel Movements: A characteristic of a healthy digestive system, promoting comfortable and predictable elimination of waste.

Reintroduction Phase: The phase where high-FODMAP foods are systematically reintroduced to identify specific carbohydrates causing symptoms.

Rome IV Diagnostic Criteria: A set of guidelines used by healthcare professionals to diagnose functional gastrointestinal disorders, including IBS.

Small Intestinal Bacterial Overgrowth (SIBO): A condition characterized by an abnormal increase in the number and/or type of bacteria in the small intestine.

Support System: A network of individuals, including friends, family, healthcare professionals, and support groups, providing encouragement and assistance during the Low FODMAP journey.

Scan this QR code to get your BONUS !

THANK YOU

Dear Valued Reader,

I hope this book has provided you with valuable insights and guidance. If it has benefited you, please consider leaving a review on Amazon. Your feedback is not only appreciated but also aids others in discovering and benefiting from this work. Thank you for your support and for being part of this journey.

Index

Mango and Lime Sorbet; 97
Mango Pineapple Mint Smoothie; 117
Mango Salsa; 110
Maple Cinnamon Roasted Nuts; 93
Maple Dijon Dressing; 107
Maple Glazed Salmon with Roasted Brussels Spr...; 66
Maple Pecan Granola with Lactose-Free Yogurt; 41
Mediterranean Baked Cod; 62
Mediterranean Chicken Skillet; 72
Mediterranean Quinoa Salad; 89
Mediterranean Stuffed Bell Peppers; 47
Nut and Seed Bars; 99
Olive Tapenade; 109
Omelet with Bell Peppers and Goat Cheese; 34
Orange Basil Mocktail; 120
Orange Ginger Turmeric Smoothie; 42
Orange Slices with Tajin; 92
Pan-Seared Steak with Chimichurri Sauce; 67
Papaya and Lime Breakfast Boat; 43
Papaya Lime Splash; 118
Peanut Butter Banana Toast; 35
Peanut Butter Energy Bites; 94
Pesto Zoodle Bowl with Cherry Tomatoes; 55
Pesto Zucchini Noodles with Grilled Chicken; 68
Pineapple Coconut Chia Pudding; 100
Pineapple Ginger Turmeric Juice; 114
Pineapple Mango Smoothie Bowl; 37
Polenta and Vegetable Breakfast Skillet; 31
Popcorn with Olive Oil and Herbs; 95
Pork and Pineapple Skewers; 61
Potato Leek Soup; 81
Potato Salad with Dijon Dressing; 87
Pumpkin and Turmeric Soup; 78
Quiche with Spinach and Lactose-Free Cheese; 37
Quinoa and Grilled Chicken Bowl; 44
Quinoa and Roasted Vegetable Salad; 83
Quinoa and Vegetable Minestrone; 76
Quinoa Breakfast Bowl with Berries; 29
Quinoa Salad with Roasted Vegetables; 52
Quinoa Tabouleh; 85
Raspberry Almond Thumbprint Cookies; 103
Ratatouille with Herbed Quinoa; 60
Red Pepper and Tomato Soup; 77
Rice Cake with Avocado and Cherry Tomatoes; 101
Rice Cake with Peanut Butter and Banana; 91

Rice Cake with Smoked Turkey and Tomato; 40
Rice Crackers with Smoked Salmon; 96
Roasted Brussels Sprouts with Bacon; 82
Roasted Chickpeas with Paprika; 99
Roasted Eggplant Soup; 79
Roasted Red Pepper & Goat Cheese Stuffed Chick..; 56
Roasted Sweet Potato Wedges; 85
Roasted Vegetable and Quinoa Casserole; 71
Salmon and Avocado Sushi Rolls; 47
Scrambled Eggs with Spinach and Tomatoes; 29
Seared Scallops with Garlic Butter; 71
Seared Tofu with Peanut Sauce; 57
Shrimp and Avocado Salad; 49
Shrimp and Mango Lettuce Wraps; 54
Shrimp Scampi with Zucchini Noodles; 62
Smoked Salmon and Avocado Wrap; 30
Spaghetti Squash with Tomato Basil Sauce; 68
Spinach and Feta Breakfast Wrap; 42
Spinach and Feta Stuffed Chicken Breast; 48
Spinach and Potato Soup; 77
Spinach and Strawberry Salad with Almonds; 88
Spinach and Tomato Breakfast Quesadilla; 34
Strawberry and Kiwi Popsicles; 98
Strawberry Balsamic Reduction; 111
Strawberry Kiwi Cooler; 114
Stuffed Acorn Squash with Quinoa and Cranberries; 69
Sweet Potato Hash with Poached Eggs; 35
Tahini Yogurt Sauce; 108
Teriyaki Chicken and Vegetable Skillet; 65
Teriyaki Sauce (without garlic and onion); 106
Teriyaki Tofu and Broccoli Stir-Fry; 51
Thai Coconut Shrimp Soup; 78
Tomato Basil Soup with Lactose-Free Cream; 75
Tuna Salad with Cucumber and Olives; 45
Turkey and Cranberry Lettuce Wraps; 44
Turkey and Cranberry Quinoa Stuffed Peppers; 54
Turkey and Zucchini Burgers; 56
Tzatziki Sauce; 112
Vegetable and Rice Paper Rolls; 58
Watermelon Cucumber Refresher; 115
Zoodle Carbonara with Bacon and Peas; 64
Zucchini and Feta Omelet; 32
Zucchini and Potato Soup; 76
Zucchini and Tomato Gratin; 73
Zucchini Noodles with Pesto and Cherry Tomatoes; 49

Printed in Great Britain
by Amazon

45078055R00077